THE YOGA OF THE KATHOPANISHAD

By

SRI KRISHNA PREM

PUBLISHERS

THE ANANDA PUBLISHING HOUSE

3A LOWTHER ROAD, ALLAHABAD

·L o

PRINTED BY J. K. SHARMA AT THE ALLAHABAD
LAW JOURNAL PRESS, ALLAHABAD

TO

M. R.

BEST OF PUPILS

FOR WHOM THIS BOOK WAS WRITTEN

त्वाद‍ङ्नो भूयान्नचिकेतः प्रष्टा

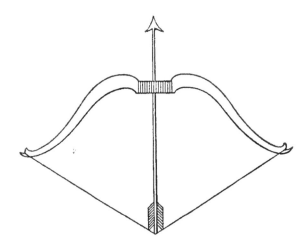

Having taken as a bow the great weapon of the Secret Teaching,
One should fix in it the arrow sharpened by constant Meditation.
Drawing it with a mind filled with That (*Brahman*)
Penetrate, O good-looking youth, that Imperishable as the Mark.

The *praṇava* (*Aum*) is the bow; the arrow is the self;
Brahman is said to be the mark.
With heedfulness is It to be penetrated;
One should become one with It as the arrow in the mark.

Muṇḍaka Upanishad ii 3, 4.

PREFACE

The point of view from which this book has been written is that the Kaṭhopanishad is a practical treatise written to help us achieve a very real end. It is not in the least a compendium of Brahmanical speculations, something to be studied from a purely intellectual viewpoint. On the contrary, it is an exposition of the ancient Road that leads from death to immortality, a Road which is as open to-day as it was when our text was written. Being a real Road the knowledge of it is not confined to any one country or to any one religious tradition. One of the aims in writing this commentary has been to bring out this fact, namely, that it is a Road known to a few all over the world and that, though their descriptions have naturally varied in detail, they all refer to what is recognisably the same experience. Previous expositions have been either from the point of view of purely Indian tradition, in terms of which alone the meanings have been set forth, or else they have been made from the artificial and external standpoint of Western scholarship which represents the teachings as being, at best, interesting religio-philosophic speculations, at worst, a tale told by an idiot, signifying nothing. With this last class of expositor it is hopeless to argue that their interpretations often make nonsense of the text for they will reply: "My dear Sir, of course it is nonsense. Why do you expect anything but the merest gleams of sense in these ancient phantasies of a childish era?" So be it. It was at least in part to hide the truth from such as these "lest having ears they should hear and be converted" that the

ancient Teachers expressed themselves so obscurely
with the aid of symbol and myth.

This brings us to another point. There will almost
certainly be those who will say of the present commentary, at least in places, that it darkens rather than
sheds light upon the text. "The text," they will say,
"was tolerably clear and straightforward, you have left
us wandering in a cloud of your incomprehensible
Black Fire ! At least you are the first (and we hope
the last) to treat the Upanishad as a text of alchemy !"

The fact is, however, that clarity (of the intellectual sort), though undoubtedly a value, is not the only
value. The true clarity which is of the Spirit is something quite different, but what is usually termed such is a
one-sided movement of mental abstraction which, like
everything one-sided, has a shadow which in this particular case appears as loss of reality. As long as we remain what we are, partial and one-sided beings, so long
each step in the direction of intellectual clarity is taken at
the cost of a loss of vividness and vitality until we arrive
in the end at the state of logic and mathematics, a state
like that of distilled water, exquisitely clear but tasteless
and sterile. On the other hand, if the archaic symbols
are left without any mental clarification the modern mind
is unable to grasp them at all and passes them by as
meaningless. Accordingly any attempt at comment
must, like any attempt at translation, be a compromise,
in this case between the degree of clarity necessary to
give any sort of clue to the meaning and the degree
of vividness coming from the sense of a rich psychic
background, necessary if the subject is to appear to
have any true reality.

Naturally the proportions of these two compo-
nents will have to vary according to conditions of time
and place. In these days there is little danger of
clarity being undervalued but rather the other way.

A previous book[1] was written with as much of it as possible. In this book, partly because it is hoped that the previous one will serve as a bridge and partly because the Upanishads have been so pawed about by intellectuals as to be in danger of being thought mere 'philosophy,' less attempt has been made to render the meaning clear to the mind. Whether the complementary value of psychic vividness has been achieved is for others to judge. If I have at all succeeded in conveying the impression that behind the words of the Upanishad lies, not a world of thin philosophic abstractions, but a world of rich and vivid experience, I shall be satisfied. "Grey is all theory, green grows the Tree of Life alone."[2]

To those who object to the alchemy I will quote Lallā, the 14th century Kashmiri Yogini:—

"Like a blacksmith give breath to the Bellows and thy Iron will turn to Gold. Now is the auspicious moment. Seek then the Friend."

Metaphor? Perhaps, but what else is the Universe?
Lastly, for those who find this book full of insufferable nonsense here is some more:—

"There was an old man of Liskeard
Who said it is just as I feared,
Five owls and a wren,
Three ducks and a hen,
Have all made their nests in my beard."

Nonsense or not, those birds are there and not the cleanest of shaves with the latest and most scientific of Occam razors will get rid of them. For *that* the only instrument that will serve is the razor-edged Middle

[1] *The Yoga of the Bhagavatgita.*
[2] Goethe's *Faust.*

Path. As for the birds, they are shape-changers. Sometimes they dazzle our senses with a flutter of tropical plumage; sometimes, as hens, they lay us useful though sulphurous eggs; sometimes, as owls they teach us wisdom of their round-eyed sort; just now on raven wings they croak above the battlefields. All these shapes are but forms of the one bird, the ugly duckling who must be led along the Middle Path from the Lower to the Upper Waters before he can assume his true Royal shape, the shape of the Eternal Swan.

"Sweet is rest between the wings of that which is not born nor dies, but is the *Aum* throughout eternal ages. Bestride the Bird of Life if thou wouldst know."

Procul este profani; Flee hence—O Academics!

CONTENTS

Contents

INTRODUCTORY NOTE

The germ of this Upanishad (to adopt a modern fashion of speaking) is to be found in a hymn in the Rig-veda (X. 135) concerning a boy, whom the commentator Sayana declares to be Nachiketas, who visits the realm of Yama, Lord of Death.

"Thou mountest though thou dost not see, O Child, the new and wheelless Vehicle which thou hast fashioned mentally, one-poled but turning every way."

In this verse we have a clear reference to the ascent of the disembodied 'Soul' in its mental *Upādhi* or vehicle. Much of the hymn is somewhat obscure. A clearer treatment is contained in the Taittirīya Brāhmaṇa (3. 11. 8, 1-6) where we have the story of the visit to Yama and the three boons granted by the latter as in our Upanishad. From the point of view of ordinary scholarship the situation is one in which this old and traditional story has been made to serve as the vehicle of Vedāntic Philosophising; but a truer way of looking at it is to consider the later text as an expression in the new language, the language of conceptual thought and more or less abstract symbolism, of the teachings which had previously been rendered in the older and more universal language of concrete symbol. This difference between the languages of concrete and of abstract symbol is a very important subject and one which requires separate treatment, but it may here be stated briefly that the philosophical teachings of all the older races, Sumerians, Egyptians, and ancient Indians, were imparted by means of concrete symbols, a method which · in spite of disadvantages, some real and some only apparent to us who have more or less lost the art of reading such symbols, has one great advantage, namely, of fusing together thought and feeling in one unity.

It seems to have been somewhere in the middle of the 1st millennium B.C., the period of the Buddha and the Upanishads, of the Hermetic writings in Egypt (in something like the form in which we know them now) and the Pythagorean-Platonic movement in Greece that the abstract symbols which we now think of as philosophic *par excellence* were developed, and came to the fore on account of their great flexibility and ease of manipulation. These qualities, however, were purchased at the cost of more or less of a divorce from feeling, a divorce which tended more and more to separate the domains of religion with its concrete symbols (Myths) and philosophy with its abstract concepts. Speaking roughly, the process may be said to have begun (in the West) in the Academy of Plato where, however, it was blended with the concrete symbols of his famous 'Myths', and to have culminated in the grey sterility of modern 'academic' thought.

CHAPTER I

(1) *Once Vājashravasa, desirous of heavenly reward, gave away all his possessions. He had a son named Nachiketas.*

(2) *Into him, boy as he was, faith entered, while the gifts (of cattle for the priests) were being led away and he reflected.*

(3) *"To joyless realms goes he who gives such cows as these, cows which have drunk their last water, eaten their last grass, have given their last milk and who will breed no more."*

(4) *Therefore he said to his father once, twice and thrice: "To whom will you give me (who also am one of your possessions)?" Whereupon the father replied, "To Death do I give thee."*

Who and what are these two, this father and son? Tradition, as exemplified by Shankara explains the name Vājashravasa as one who is famous for his gifts of food *or*, as he says, the compound may be just a proper name. The 'or' here reveals the fact that Shankara was aware that such names in the ancient myths were by no means mere names but that they often, if not always, carried meanings which are of great importance in the understanding of the myths. We are reminded of the Egyptian Book of the Dead as also of the Indian Kaushītaki Upanishad in which the soul on its inward path is confronted by various symbolic objects, doorways, trees and such like, which will not let it pass unless it reveals its knowledge of their 'Names.'

In just the same way, these ancient myths (the psychic as opposed to the mere mental reading of which constitutes an initiation) confront us at the outset with names whose inner meanings we must apprehend under penalty of complete failure to enter the sacred precincts. It is just this fact that is the reason for so much of the apparently fanciful etymologising of which modern scholars accuse the ancient writers. So-called fanciful derivations, based as they often are on associations, are frequently of more real significance in these mystic realms than all the great tomes of carefully accurate but sterile learning.[1]

Vājashravasa is composed of two words *Vāja* and *Shravasa* of which it is quite true that the former means food and the latter fame. But these are only particular applications, special readings, as it were of the far more inclusive original symbols. *Vāja*, for instance, only means food because food increases the "strength, energy spirit, speed" which are some of its more fundamental meanings. The feather on an arrow again is also *Vāja* while *Shravasa* means fundamentally a loud sound, something which is heard—whence fame as a derivative.

In this context the word *Vājashravasa* refers to what

---

[1] Just before going to press my friend Thakur Jaideva Singhji sent me a set of Dr. A. Coomaraswami's *Notes on the Kaṭhopanishad* which appeared in the *New Indian Antiquary* for April, May, and June 1938. They arrived too late to be made any extensive use of but some footnote references to them have been inserted. These 'Notes' will very well repay study as their learned author has at his command a depth and breadth of scholarship which the present writer cannot hope to compass and, moreover, what is so rare as to be almost unique in the world of modern scholarship, he takes the Upanishad seriously as a Gnostic document related as such to Gnostic literature all over the world. It should be added, however, that they are addressed to students with a knowledge of Sanskrit. In the present context he cites Rawson as saying: "probably the names which are all patronymics are not meant to be historical."

may be called exoteric religion, the tradition about the *sustaining power* of the Universe which has been *heard* and handed down through generations. It is as a symbol of such exoteric religion that the man Vājashravasa speaks and acts.

The name of the son, Nachiketas, on the other hand, is derived from *na chiketas*, that which is unperceived and refers to the quickening Spirit that lies within all things like fire, latent in wood, "hidden in the two fire sticks," unperceived by the senses and yet the spirit which giveth life as opposed to Vājashravasa, the letter which killeth.

Vājashravasa, then, represents orthodox traditional religion, devoted as always to outer forms, ignorant of the real meaning of which those forms are the vehicles, content with their literal observance, and wise like all traditionalist priests, Hindu or Catholic, in the knowledge of backdoors and short cuts by which the forms may be preserved without too great an inconvenience in practice!

Sacrifice and gifts are commanded by tradition and therefore Vājashravasa, forgetful of what is meant by that sacrifice, gives away his possessions with considerable ostentation, but, finding such giving not altogether convenient, compromises somehow and makes a great show of a lot of rather inadequate cows.

As actual facts such performances are common in India and of course everywhere else, but in the present case the meaning is not particular but universal. It is the externalism, not to say hypocrisy, inherent in all exoteric religion that is referred to, rather than individual acts of religious compromise.

Nevertheless, a genuine religious tradition, though externalised into more or less sterile forms, is not to be despised. That is the mistake of the so-called rationalists. Neither religion nor life itself is, has been or ever will be a matter of reason alone. Religion springs from the depth of the psyche and its rational elements are only part of its total content. Not only the 'rationalist,' but also the protestant type of reformer, is apt to make this mistake and, in rationalising religion, to render it sterile. For instance in India there are some people who do not like the rowdy horse-play, not to say the verbal license, which characterises the ancient festival of Holi and they wish to substitute a day of quiet meditation on the birth of Chaitanya which happened to coincide with the festival. Such quiet meditation is certainly excellent, but it just isn't Holi, and in making such a substitution the deep psychic meanings of the ancient festival are entirely lost.

This, however, is a digression. Within the heart of the old traditions, if they be not too utterly dead, there comes to birth from time to time a son who is a re-birth of the ancient ever-living Spirit which gave rise to the religion.

Such a son is Nachiketas. He is the new born Spirit, ever breathing the Upanishadic prayer "From the unreal lead me to the Real." Such births as actual individual events are continually taking place at all times and then we have a mystic, one who seeks to pierce through the outer veil and re-enter the deserted inner sanctuary. Such a man becomes a disciple of the Inner Path and therefore we have Nachiketas, standing first as a symbol of the reborn Spirit which slumbers in the heart of all religions, and secondly as a glyph of the individual mystic, he who seeks out and treads the "Ancient narrow path that stretches far away."[1] It is particularly in this latter sense that we shall read the symbol here.

Into his heart, we read, faith (*Shraddhā*), entered.

[1] Brihadāranyaka Upanishad 4. 4. 8.

Chapter I

This *Shraddhā* is never to be confounded with what passes for faith in the exoteric religion, namely, a blind belief, accompanied, as is all such, by hidden doubt. In this latter sense *Vājashravasa* himself had faith, or else why did he perform the sacrifice at all? but it is a faith which is balanced by equal and opposite concealed doubts: the faith of all exoteric religion which hopes and at the same time fears. The *Shraddhā* which entered Nachiketas is the true faith, the Fair Faith as Hermes calls it, which is a form of knowledge, being the reflection in the personal self of Knowledge that has been realised at deeper levels of being. In technical terms it is the reflection in the personal mind of the Knowledge that results from the union of the higher *manas* with the *buddhi*. For the personal mind it is not quite knowledge, because that personal or lower mind is not yet properly united to its higher self, and therefore the latter's Knowledge can only appear as the reflection which we term faith.

The transmutation of such faith into Knowledge is indeed the task which the disciple will have to perform, the Path which he must tread. Nevertheless, though as yet only a reflection, it is reflection of the Truth and if he clings to it as to a guiding star, "the dim star which burns within," it will transmute his whole being into the divine solar light of perfect Knowledge.

"Steadily as you watch and worship its light will grow stronger. Then you may know you have found the beginning of the way. And when you have found the end its light will suddenly become the infinite light."[1]

It is by the light of this faith that Nachiketas realises the inadequacy of all mere outward forms. The true sacrifice, though it may be usefully embodied in forms, is the sacrifice of the self and it is just this that

[1] *Light on the Path.*

2

Vājashravasa withholds. Hence the protest implied in his son's question. I who am also your possession, the most valued one in fact, your very self, to whom will you give me ? To whom am I, the spirit born of your heart, to be offered ? Nor does the question spring from the mind alone but from the whole of his being, hence its triple repetition for man is a citizen of three worlds and must ask and be willing for the sacrifice on every level of his being.[1]

"Those that ask shall have. But though the ordinary man asks perpetually his voice is not heard. For he asks with his mind only; and the voice of the mind is only heard on that plane on which the mind acts."[2]

It is this threefold integration of man's being that is the real root of such current feelings as of the sacred and binding quality of a threefold affirmation, the 'third time of asking,' that is found in one form or another all over the world.

"To Death do I give you." These are the solemn words which are pronounced when the offer is complete. One well-known Christian missionary translator considers these tremendous words to have been pronounced in mere irritation and suggests that they might be rendered as, "Oh ! go to Hades !" Did he not remember Christ's "Ye must be born again" and is it not obvious that before we can be reborn we must first die ? To all such we will only quote their Teacher's words. "Art thou a master of Israel and knowest not these things ?" Do we not die every night to be reborn next day ? Does not the very Sun himself die every year to be reborn at the X'mas solstice and is it not true that, as

---

[1] Those who know the Sanyāsa mantra will remember how the Sanyāsi renounces the world of forms not only on this but on all three levels *Bhū, Bhuvar, Swar.*

[2] *Light on the Path.*

St. Paul has it: "Thou fool, that which thou sowest is not quickened except it die."[1]

Leaving controversy aside, let us turn to that fragment of ancient initiatory teaching that is known as the Naasene Document.

"The Phrygians call Him (Man) also Dead—when buried in the body as though in a tomb or a sepulchre... ...The same Phrygians again call this very same (Man) after the transformation God or a God......and they call him also "Plucked Green Wheat Ear" and after the Phrygians, the Athenians (so designate Him) when in the secret rites at Eleusis, they show those who receive in silence the final initiation there into the Great Epoptic mystery, a plucked wheat ear. And the wheat ear is also with the Athenians the Light Giver from the Inexpressible. And the law is that after they have been initiated into the Little Mysteries they should be further initiated into the Great. 'For greater Deaths do greater lots obtain,' (and) they to whom 'Deaths' in them (the Greater Mysteries) are appointed receive greater lots."[2]

This is the same eternal wisdom, the wisdom that teaches us that if we would find our true life we must first lose the false one that is lived in the sunlight of the world and take the other Path, "death-cold" to sense, but leading to the true Sunlight of Eternity, for as we may remember from the Gita: "that which is Day to

---

[1] Cf. Coomarswamy—"Hume's paraphrase of the Father's words, e. g., 'Oh! go to Hades' is bad enough, but far more shocking is Rawson's 'His father, however, angered by the persistence of his priggish son buts forth with the equivalent of an angry Englishman's 'Go to hell !' ' With the angry Englishman we are only too familiar: his introduction here is a profanity."

[2] The quotations are from G. R. S. Mead's version in *Thrice Greatest Hermes* I, 148, et seq., omitting the interpolations of another, though, allied school. The Naasenes were the followers of Naas, the serpent or Dragon of Wisdom.

the many is Night to the Seer and that which is Day to the seer is Night to the ordinary man."

The mystic death which played an essential part in all the ancient rites of initiation is in fact the gate through which must pass all who seek the light of wisdom. Psychologists will explain it in terms of introversion and ethical writers in those of self-abnegation and what they write will be all quite true. It is these things but it is also very much more for here, as always, the ancient symbols have a wealth of content to which it is impossible to do full justice with our modern conceptual thought. The Mystic Death is a real death and, like all that is real, it has its dangers. We know that candidates were often terrified during the process of initiation both in Greece and elsewhere and Tibetan gurus of the so-called Direct Path warn their pupils that they run three grave risks—illness, madness and (literal) death. It has also been said that "he who would cross the threshold of any world must leave fear behind him."[1] Here, however, let us return to our text. Those who seek the Mystic Death will assuredly find it if they ask for it "Three Times."

Once embarked on this path Nachiketas reflects within his heart.

(5) *Of many I go as the first (and yet) of many I am in the midst. What is the task that Yama, Lord of Death, will accomplish on me today?*

(6) *Bear in mind how went those who have gone before. Note how in the same way go others now. Like grain a mortal ripens and like grain is he born again.*

One of the characteristics of the ordeal through which Nachiketas has to pass, a characteristic that has

[1] *Lilith* by George Macdonald.

been noted by so many of those who have left any record of their passing, is the sense of loneliness that accompanies it. Just as he who dies physically has to leave behind all possessions, all friends, and all relations, even the dearest, so does the candidate on this inner path have to leave behind all the ties he has contracted, to sever all the links that bind him to the life he now leaves behind for ever, and voyage on alone. But this is not all. The teachers who have so far guided him along the Path can take him no further while that Teacher "who is to give thee birth in the Hall of Wisdom, the Hall which lies beyond,"[1] has either not yet shown his face or else has for the time withdrawn it from the disciple's vision. Not that he has really withdrawn. In reality He is ever at the side of his spiritual son but it is an immutable law that the latter must pass alone through this ordeal, seemingly unaided, and relying solely on his own inner strength.

Hence, at this point, Nachiketas, in his loneliness can only seek strength within by reflection that he is but one of a chain, that many have safely made the passage before and that others are even now doing so. What has been done by man, man can do again. So without regrets for that past life towards which, if one looks back, he is lost, he prepares himself for the mystic journey by reflecting on its significance so that he may make it in full consciousness instead of having to pass through a dark belt of unconsciousness such as is passed through in the involuntary death of the ordinary man.

"Easy is the descent into the World of Death! But to retrace one's steps ! That is the task, that the labour !"[2] This ability to retrace one's steps, to bring back into this world the secret knowledge gained Be-

---

[1] *Voice of the Silence.*

[2] *Aeneid* VI.

yond, it is this that above all characterises the voluntary death of the Initiate and distinguishes it from the physical death which comes to all men and also from the death-like trance of the mere passive medium.

None can confer this power on him who is not able to find it in himself. Out of the depths of our own being must come the strength that is to carry us over the barrier. Reflecting, therefore, on the fact that his predecessors on the Path have successfully achieved the journey, Nachiketas reminds himself also of the fact that such death and rebirth is the great law of the Cosmos.

Once more we have this famous Corn, the grain of St. Paul's teachings already quoted, the Plucked Wheat Ear of the Greek (Eleusinian) Mysteries, the Corn seven cubits high of the Egyptian Fields of Aahlu.

Modern man is only too ready to consider all this as mere irrelevant metaphor, of no serious importance in a discussion of what he calls the problem of survival. He marvels that anyone can have derived comfort from what, if it is not what he calls a 'fertility Myth,' is mere analogy and (to him) not a very good one at that. Surely his God has sealed up his eyes and ears "lest having eyes he should see and having ears understand." To him the sacred Plucked Wheat Ear may be nothing but an ear of wheat, but to him who trod, as to him who now treads, the ancient Path it is no mere *triticum vulgare* but the "Great, marvellous, and most perfect Mystery of Initiation, the Light Giver from That which is Inexpressible," That which is the Darkness beyond all light. He who, having passed through the proper training and discipline, gazes on the mysterious Wheat Ear finds in it a window through which he can gaze deep into the inner World of Causes and see there the realities which underlie this outer world of appearances and effects. It was not mere

Chapter I

faith, based on childish reasoning by analogy, that gave strength of soul to the ancient initiates, and, as we know from the testimony of Greek writers even in those later days when the Mysteries were in decline, conferred on them *knowledge* of their own immortality. Almost alone among the academic moderns, the philosopher Whitehead seems, with his doctrine of universal prehensions, to be within measurable distance of understanding how each point in the universe apprehends all other points and how it is thus possible to see "Infinity in a grain of sand."[1] It is useless to say more. Those who have seen the Wheat Ear will understand what is meant: those who have not will never be able to see anything more than *triticum vulgare* and unsound analogy.

Note, however, that even at this stage, Nachiketas is perfectly aware that after death, like corn, we are born again; in other words, that death is not the end and that re-incarnation is a law of nature. The importance of this will be seen later.

Something, however, must be said of Yama, the Lord of Death, whose name is mentioned in verse five. The name itself has several meanings, most fundamental of which appears to be the idea of checking and restraining, as with a bridle (whence *Yama* the first branch of eightfold Yoga). It is also important to note that it means a twin and in the Vedic symbolism Yama has a twin sister Yami.[2] In the Rigveda,[3] these two speak of themselves as "the children of Gandharva and the Water-nymph, in other words, as born of the intercourse of the Spirit of Harmony, the *Buddhi*, above and the Spirit of Water,

[1] Blake.
[2] We may also note the parallel with Yima and Yimeh, who in the Avestan tradition, were the primaeval twins who produced the human race.
[3] Rv., X 10. 4. quoted by Macdonell.

23

the lower world of 'Matter' and desire. It is in this sense that we have to read the hymn which relates Yami's consuming passion for her twin brother. In another hymn (X. 14) Yama is spoken of as the first "who travelled to the lofty heights above us, who searches out and shows the path to many, Yama first found for us a place to dwell in; this pasture never can be taken from us." The imaginary first man who died, say the scholars. Doubtless; but, at least in this context, what sort of 'death' is it with which we are concerned? Others, however, are nearer the mark for we have E. Meyer saying that Yama is the *alter ego*, the other Self of man. The actual nature of the Path he discovered is shown clearly enough in the previous hymn X. 13. "Five paces (the five levels of consciousness) have I risen from the Earth......This by the sacred Syllable ('The Om, the divisions of which measure the worlds, see *Māndukya Upanishad*) have I measured: I purify (the Soma, the drops of which signify the process of individuali-sation) in the central place of Order (the central point between the two inverted triangles ⧗)."

The fact is that Yama is the individual soul, the higher *manas* with his twin sister, the lower or personal mind. That is why the pair are born between the Harmony above and the Desire nature beneath; why also, according to a different myth, that is referred to in our Upanishad, he is Vaivaswata, son of the Sun and so is equivalent to Manu who also is a symbol of the central point, the microcosm, the little Sun of the true Individuality. Hence, he is depicted[1] as green in colour, clothed in red and riding on a buffalo, the symbol of the lower nature, tamed and made into a ve-hicle for the higher. He is the inner controller, the Voice of true conscience, ("the fear of death !") and

[1] See Monier Williams' Sanskrit Dictionary.

Chapter 1

elsewhere has been described as dwelling in a palace made of iron and copper. Those who are aware of the symbolic meanings of the various colours and metals will be able from the above description alone to understand His nature.

Exoterically he is, like the Greek Minos, the Judge of the dead, but this of course only confirms the interpretation given above, for it is by man himself that man's acts are judged and he who judges us is not any external power but, as stated in the twelfth chapter of Manu, our higher Self. That he should seem to most men a sinister and menacing figure is the inevitable consequence of the fact referred to in the Gita that "the Self is the friend of the self and the same Self is the enemy of the self. It is the friend of him whose (lower) self is mastered but to the uncontrolled (lower) self the Self manifests as a veritable enemy."[1]

It is thus that, to the ordinary man, Yama appears as the grim Judge, while, to the disciple of the inner Path who has controlled and harmonised his lower mind it is not as Judge but as the great Initiator, "he who will give thee birth in the Hall of Wisdom," that he manifests. It is, as we shall see in this guise that he appears to Nachiketas.

Nachiketas then undertakes the journey, the Death that Eugenius Philalethes well calls "a regress into the hiddenness," and travelling along that inner Path whose gateway is in the heart, arrives at the Halls of Yama, where, however, he at first finds naught but emptiness. In that mystic Emptiness an impersonal Voice is heard setting forth one of the universal laws of life.

(7) *As a very fire, the Brāhman guest enters into houses, therefore, O Son of the Sun, bring water to assuage him.*

[1] Gita VI 5 and 6.

The text goes on to add an explanation of this somewhat cryptic utterance.

(8) *Hope and expectation, friendly intercourse, the merits gained by sacrifice and charitable acts, offspring and cattle—for the foolish man in whose house a Brāhman (guest) has to fast all these things are destroyed.*

The Hindus, like all other ancient peoples, have always attached great importance to the hospitable treatment of the stranger who comes within their doors and innumerable precepts lay down that a stranger guest is to be considered as a god and treated as such. Especially is this the case when the guest is a man of learning and austere life—such as were the Brāhmans in ancient times. Such a man, coming unasked to one's house, is a great blessing and to slight his advent or to fail to show him respect is an act which is fraught with grave consequences. This fact is one which was known to all the ancient peoples, to primitive tribes at the present day and to all who have not sold their psychic birthright for a mess of mental pottage. A magic mantle is always on the shoulders of the Stranger and therefore he is always a potential danger if not properly and hospitably received. "As a fire he enters the house." Moreover, the word used for fire in this verse is not that used for the everyday fire of the hearth but Vaishvānara, the Universal Fire, that which is 'common to all men,' the great Fire, which is the unity of all life. It is because he comes as an embodiment of this ultimate unity and not as a mere bearer of those ties of relationship which we ourselves create and project on our surroundings, that the opportunity of serving the Stranger Guest is so golden a one for us, and that the slighting of him, a slight against the very Spirit of Life, is fraught with such serious consequences.

Chapter I

The water which Yama, Son of the Sun, is asked to fetch is the water for washing the feet, which is the first offering made by Hindus, whether to Gods or guests.

In all this, however, we are still only dealing with the outer garments of our text. A deeper insight is afforded by the words of *Light on the Path*. "When the disciple is ready to learn, then he is accepted, acknowledged, recognised. It must be so, for he has lit his lamp and it cannot be hidden." Also by those of the *Voice of the Silence*: "Not one recruit can ever be refused the right to enter on the Path that leads to the field of Battle."

Nachiketas remains for three nights in the Halls of Yama without the latter putting in an appearance. He now appears and says:

(9) *O Brahman, you, a worshipful guest, have dwelt for three nights foodless in my house. Therefore I offer you my reverence. Choose in return three boons (and) may it be well for me.*

Nachiketas has entered on the Path, he has 'lit his lamp' and its golden flame is burning steadily in the 'windless place' of the Emptiness within. The candidates in ancient initiations had to remain for three days and three nights in a death-trance, awaiting the mystic rebirth and Christ remained for the same time in the tomb during which period he descended to the Underworld, the Realm of Death. Nachiketas too has remained for three nights in the inner Emptiness of Yama's Halls and the bright flame of his lamp, now undisturbed by the winds of desire, is bound to attract the attention of his higher self, personified by Yama. "When the disciple is ready the Master appears." At this point the teacher in *Light on the Path* says, almost

in the same words as the Upanishad: "Peace be with
you" and goes on to add the teaching.
"Regard the three truths. They are equal."
The coincidence of this with the three boons of our
text is remarkable or, rather, would be so if it were not
for the fact that both these treatises come from the same
source and consequently are bound to be in agree-
ment.

Before we pass on we should note that a deep significance attaches to the fact that Nachiketas ate no food
in the Halls of Death. We may remember the myth
of the Rape of Persephone by Pluto, Lord of the
Dead, and how her complete return to the upper
world was hindered by the fact that she had eaten a
pomegranate seed in those underworld halls. Also
how, in Celtic folklore, he who enters the underground
palaces of the fairies must, if he would return thence
to his friends in the world, abstain carefully from
eating anything. To eat the food of any plane of
being is to assimilate oneself thereto and the candidate who essays the dangerous journey to the inner
planes must be careful to 'fast,' to retain his roots in
this plane of consciousness, to exercise a vigilant
self-control or self-recollectedness, if he wishes to be
able to return thence with the wisdom he has garnered.
If for a moment he loses hold, if he allows himself
to be carried away and be assimilated to the existence
there, the link which binds him to his physical body
will be snapped and the Path of return be closed until
in the normal way of reincarnation he treads it once
more into a new body.

We shall now pass on to the first of Nachiketas'
three boons.

(10) *As the first of the three boons I choose that when
sent back by thee, O Death, my father Gautama, his sacri-*

*ficial intent accomplished, may recognise and welcome me with
a mind peaceful and free from the fiery turmoil of the heart.*

To which Yama replies:

(11) *As aforetime will that son of ancient Sages[1]
behave towards thee. Having seen thee liberated from the
mouth of Death and recognising thee as one sent back by Me[2]
he will sleep happily of nights, his turmoil stilled.*

The literal meaning of these verses is of course
quite clear. Nachiketas prays that when he returns to
the world his father may recognise him and not cast
him off in fear (as has happened quite often to those
who have returned to their homes after an apparent
physical death) and that the turmoil of heart in which
the father had despatched his son to death may be al-
layed. We may notice, in passing, a touch of the Odys-
seus-like cunning with which the typical hero of folklore is always endowed. Nachiketas does not ask directly that he may be allowed to return, but skilfully
enough inserts *that* boon within the structure of a
wider one.

Underneath this natural human wish, however,
lie, as usual, far deeper meanings. We have seen that
Vājashravasa typifies the orthodox and exoteric reli-

[1] The actual phrase is Auddālaki Āruṇi, a patronymic of
Vājashravasa, Uddalaka and Aruṇa being ancient sages. As,
however, Auddālaki also means a kind of honey produced by bees
who live in the earth and Aruṇa was the charioteer of the Sun,
we might render it as 'that Earth-born son of the Morning
Twilight,' a very appropriate title for one who symbolises
the ancient religious traditions descending from the Cosmic
Dawn.

[2] There is some scholarly fuss about the grammatical case
of *prasrishṭaḥ* but the general sense is quite clear.

gious traditions. The attitude of all such towards those sons of their bosom who venture forth along the mystic paths and return thence with new wisdom has always been a somewhat doubtful one. In mediaeval Catholicism the 'holy' Inquisition was always liable to be asked to sit in judgment on the new wisdom which her mystics brought and woe to the latter if the Church decided that the new wine was too dangerous to be contained in the old bottles. Such brutalities as resulted in Europe were scarcely, if at all, known in the gentler and wiser (gentler *because* wiser) psyche of India, with its unparalleled power of assimilating the new without ruining the structure of the old. Nevertheless, it is always an anxious moment for the mystic when, returning with his hands laden with gifts, he wonders what sort of a welcome he is to receive. Nor is this anxiety as to his reception by any means founded on selfish considerations. It is of the greatest importance that the new life which he brings shall be able to be grafted successfully on to the old tree otherwise the toils and ordeals of his pilgrimage will have been undergone in vain—not for himself—whom nothing earthly can touch—but for the world. In recent times we have seen how one of the greatest of such Initiates, H. P. Blavatsky, was received on her return. Slander and vilification met her everywhere and it was only with the most superhuman exertions, coupled with the 'boon of Yama,' that she was able to prevent her richly laded vessel from being overturned and its contents all spilled in the stormy turmoil that her coming raised. Assuredly it was no light or superficial request, no mere edifying piece of filial piety, that Nachiketas chose when, as the first of his boons, he prayed that the old tradition, descended from the ancient Teachers of the Dawn, should welcome back with open arms him whom it had sent forth.

Chapter I

We now come to the second boon.

(12) *In the Heaven World there is no fear. Thou (death) art not there nor does one fear old age. Having passed beyond both of these,. as also beyond hunger and thirst, the Sorrowless Ones there in that Heaven rejoice.*

(13) *Thou, O Death, knowest that Fire by which the Heaven Dwellers attain immortality; teach it to me, therefore, who am full of faith. This I choose as my second boon.*

Nachiketas' second request is for knowledge of the Heavenly Fire, the Sacred Fire of the alchemists by which the lead of the personal self is transmuted into the Gold of the (relatively) immortal Higher Ego. The Vedic tradition had taught that by various kinds of offering in fire, man could attain the spacious Heaven World, such attainment being, as always with exoteric religions, deferred till after the death of the body. Those who performed the correct sacrifices—and their absolute correctness was held to be of great importance— after the death of the physical body, went to dwell in the wide plains of Heaven, whose very name of *Swarloka* indicates their nature as the true home of the higher Self. It is there that true individuality has its being, there that it dwells. From time to time it sends forth its projected images into the lower world of birth and death and those images are our personal selves. They are thrown down into the Sea of physical matter like a fisher's nets, and, when their 'catch' of experience is full, they are withdrawn once more by the Fisher. He himself does not descend into the Sea but sits above in his boat throughout the long ages of the Cosmic Day, knowing in himself neither birth nor death nor sorrow. Therefore is he said to be immortal, though truly endless he is not, for he is a part of the manifested universe and all that is manifest must sooner or later return into That from which it emerged.

Nevertheless, his 'duration' is incalculable as we count time for he endures, as the old alchemists were fond of saying, as long as Nature itself. The safe re-union of the projected personality with that Ego which had sent it forth, a union to be attained after death constituted the goal of the exoteric Vedic religion, as it has constituted that of *all* exoteric religions. We have said the safe re-union. It might be thought that, the situation being as stated above, such reunion after death was inevitable and in the nature of things, so that there would be no need to do anything special about it. This, however, is not so. To return to our symbol of the Fisher, the net may break while being hauled up or its catch may be of a nature that is uneatable by the Fisher and so is thrown away. In other words, the personal self, endowed as it is with a measure of the divine free-will of its projector, may use that will to break away altogether; or, more often, its catch of experience may be of such a nature (what we know as evil deeds) that it is unassimilable by the higher Self and therefore has to be thrown away. In such a case the Fisher himself remains what he always was, immortal, but the personal self, failing to achieve union, perishes and dies in what St. Paul termed the second death. If, however, the re-union is safely achieved, the personal self dwells blissfully within the bosom of its Father, sharing in the latter's immortality until, after a period which may extend to many many centuries, his garnered experiences are fully assimilated and he merges blissfully into the being of the Fisher, who thereupon sends forth a new projection which shall be heir to the deeds of its predecessor. In our crude terms he is born again down here, though exactly who or what is born again is a question which, as the Buddhists found, is easier to ask than to answer.

Such union *after death*, with its long period of un-trammelled heavenly bliss, has always been, we repeat, the goal of exoteric religion. In all countries, however, and at all times, there have been a few who were aware that more than this could be achieved. In all parts of the world there have been the persistent traditions of the *Chiranjivas*, the Undying Ones, the Sons who have become one with their Fathers and who have attained, *while here on earth*, a state of permanent union with their Higher Selves. The lives of such Men are quite beyond our comprehension. Living and perhaps wandering about in the world, to all appearance like ordinary mortals, they have passed through the *Mystic Death* and what can be seen by us is only their outer shadow, for the centre of their being is firmly rooted in those higher Selves with which they are in complete union and from which they live. Their physical forms are conscious and willed images or projections over which they exercise complete control, while ours are from a source of which we are not conscious and over which, therefore, we have at least a most inadequate control.

The higher Self is referred to in the Gita as *Vashi*, the controller,[1] with whom we have already seen Yama is identical. Hence it is that Nachiketas requests from Yama as his second boon, the knowledge of the Sacred Fire by which the transmutation of the mortal or leaden personal self into the immortal or golden Higher Self can be brought about here and now. There have always been a few in this world, as to this day there are, who have the knowledge of this Fire, the great secret to which the true alchemists were always referring but which they always guarded with the utmost jealousy, taking care to say nothing whatever that could be understood by the uninitiated. Nor is their reserve

[1] Gita V. 13.

in any sense a selfish desire to monopolise knowledge. The Sacred Fire, for all their talk about its "gentle natural warmth," can also manifest as destructively as the lightening flash, the *Vajra* or thunderbolt of Indra, with which it is in fact connected. He who should discover it before he is ready to hold in himself its tremendous power, he who out of curiosity or to gratify base desires, including the desire for prolongation of mere personal life, should succeed in awakening it would be as utterly destroyed as would he who should stand in the path of the lightning: for though it is the Universal Medicine, yet it can kill as readily as it can cure. It is for this reason that such secrecy about it has always been maintained. Those who seek it must do so in the Halls of Death, for only to him who is Dead while yet alive, is its secret revealed.

Yama now speaks:

(14) *Knowing that Heavenly Fire, I explain it to thee. Do thou therefore, O Nachiketas, understand it well of me. Know that that Fire, the means of the attainment of unending being, the Support or Basis of all the worlds is hidden in the Cave of the heart.*

(15) *Then He told him of that Fire which is the creative power that builds the worlds, with what kind of bricks its altar is to be made, both how many and how they are to be arranged. And Nachiketas repeated whatever was told him by Death, so that the latter, satisfied with the pupil, spoke again.*

(16) *Being pleased, the Mahātma said: here and now I give to thee another boon. In thy own name shall this Fire be known in future. Accept from me also this Garland of many forms.*

Nachiketas, having come to the Halls of Death and having, therefore, renounced all personal desire, is one who can be safely entrusted with the Knowledge to which he is indeed now entitled. Hence the Teacher explains it to him without further ado. He tells him that this Fire is the Creative Power which brings about the manifestation of all worlds, of which it is thus the Root or basis, that it is the means for attaining unending being, and that it is to be found hidden in the Cave that is within the hearts of all beings. This Fire is identical with what has been termed *Kundalini*, the Serpent Power which according to some schools dwells at the base of the spine but which is more correctly stated to have its hiding place in the 'heart.'

"Let the fiery power retire into the inmost chamber, the chamber of the Heart, and the abode of the world's Mother," says the Voice of the Silence and adds that, "before the 'mystic Power' can make of thee a god, O Lanoo, thou must have gained the faculty to slay thy lunar form at will." The 'lunar form' is of course the desire nature which must have passed through death before the Knowledge can be given or safely used. Naturally the actual instructions given by Yama about the Fire are not repeated in the text. Nor, for reasons already stated, are they given in any text known to the world. All that is stated is that an altar has to be built into which the Fire is to be invoked and that it has to be constructed in a special manner and of a particular number of bricks (*ishtakāh*). The 'bricks' are stated by Madhvāchārya to be living Powers (*Devatās*) and he gives their number as 360, the number of the year or the full circle. By a threefold subdivision of each brick the *Aitareya Brāhmana* gives the number as 1080. The present writer is in no position to disclose more and the reader must use his own intuition if he seeks to draw forth further knowledge from the text. All that can be said has been said long ago, namely, that the full Circle must be Squared and all its living Powers concentred in one Point.

The Yoga of the Kaṭhopaniṣhad

It is interesting to note that Shankara, if indeed the *bhāshya* on this Upanishad that goes by his name was really written by the great Shankara, either displays or chooses to display less insight into the meaning of this section than does Madhva, the dualist. While Shankara tends to belittle the question of the Sacred Fire as merely concerned with heavenly 'beer and skittles,' Madhva, forced as may be some of his rendering of later sections, exhibits deeper knowledge of the true meaning of these verses.

Quoting from the *Brahma Sāra*, he states that he who performs three times the Nachiketas Fire Sacrifice resides in the Heaven World for a whole Cosmic Period and thence attains final Liberation along with Brahmā himself at the end of the Day. In other words, it concerns the knowledge of what is known as *Krama-mukti* or Liberation by stages, a Path which has been much misunderstood ever since Shankara chose to belittle it in favour of the *Sadyo-mukti* or sudden and entire Liberation which was the teaching of his school.

In this matter Madhva is undoubtedly right. It is a great mistake to treat any of the three boons as trivial in importance. They correspond to what the alchemists refer to as the three aspects of the Great Work, the Philosophical, the Religious and the Metallic. As the accomplishment of the other two depends on the accomplishment of the Philosophic Work, it is the latter upon which the Upanishad dwells at length. Moreover, it is the only one which can be safely written about except in the darkest symbols.

However little or much we may understand the details of the altar etc. we have at least been given the all-important statement that the Secret Fire is hidden in our own hearts. Nachiketas repeats the teachings as a sign that he has assimilated them. Pleased with the aptness of his pupil Yama then offers, of his own ac-

36

cord, a further boon. The word *Mahātma* is used here, as it is used in the eleventh chapter of the Gita, in a very definite sense. In modern India any religious mendicant is apt to be called a Mahātma and even those who would shrink from such a usage at least take it to mean any genuinely spiritual man. Nevertheless, like the word *Maharshi*, which does not merely mean 'great Rishi,' the term *Mahātma*—literally Great Self—has definite reference to that level of being technically known as '*Mahat*,' more or less equivalent to what is known as the Soul of the World. The true Mahātmas are those who have identified their being with that Cosmic Soul and who, if they at all preserve a separate focus of individuality, such as we think of as a particular self, do so solely for the benefit of the living beings of whom they are the true Teachers and Guides. As Shankara has it: "Themselves crossed over, they remain out of compassion for men and in order to help them also to make the crossing."[1]

Yama tells Nachiketas that in future the Fire will be known in the world by his name and in fact, as we have already seen, the name *Nachiketas*, literally the unperceived, is one which refers expressly to the Hidden Fire. Just such a hidden fire is every disciple and indeed every man whatever. At the final initiation that Fire bursts into Flame, burning up all limitations so that the disciple remains a disciple no more but himself becomes a Teacher.

Nachiketas further receives a present of a garland of many forms. This Garland has more than one significance. In the first place it is the *Varṇa-mālā*, the celebrated Garland of Letters worn by the Goddess Kali and signifies the knowledge of all the hidden Powers of Nature. Secondly it refers to the series of his

[1] *Viveka Chudāmaṇi.*

previous lives which, strung together like so many
beads upon the string of the enduring Higher Self, now
become known to him. This memory of his past
lives was not indeed asked for by the disciple but it
is an inevitable result of the attainment of the stage now
reached by him. The knower of the Fire is able as we
have seen to unite his lower or personal self with
the higher and enduring one and in that Higher Self
the memories have all the time existed, just as in our
ordinary personal selves exist the memories of the
various periods which we have passed through in this
life. When the two selves are united, the entire series
of memories naturally becomes available.[1]

(17) *He who has thrice kindled the Nachiketas Fire*
(or perhaps *a triple Nachiketas Fire*), *has united with the
Three, and performed the three Acts, crosses over beyond birth
and death. Having known and thoroughly realised that Shining Power, the Knower who is born of Brahman and (who is
the one) Power deserving of worship, one goes to the
everlasting Peace.*

(18) *The wise man who having kindled the triple Nachiketas Fire and known this Triad, builds up that Fire in
meditation, he having already (that is, while still living) destroyed the bonds of death, gone beyond sorrow, enjoys the bliss
of the Heaven World.*

(19) *This is thy Heavenly Fire, O Nachiketas, which
thou hast chosen as thy second boon. After thee in truth
will this Fire be named by men. Now choose thy third boon.*

[1] Coomaraswamy paraphrases *anekarūpa* by *vishwarūpa* and
considers the garland to be the power of the divine omnifor-
mity as opposed to the one form to which the ignorant self is
limited. He quotes a Buddhist text (Majjhima 1. 387) which
reads "Just as one might weave a manifold garland, even so
in the Bhagwan (Buddha) there is full many a form (*aneka vaṇṇo*).
Yea many hundreds of forms." This interpretation varies only
very slightly if at all from that given here.

Chapter I

These three verses, which some translators have thought to be interpolations, merely implement what has been said before about the Fire. The Fire when kindled is a triple one, for it burns on all the three great levels of man's being, as represented by the Vedic terms *Bhū*, *Bhuvar* and *Swar*. It has been referred to elsewhere as the three-tongued Flame of the four Wicks. On all three levels, physical, intermediate (or astral as it is often called) and mental, the Fire must be kindled if the eccentric lower personality is to be transmuted into the higher. The Fire is one but the Furnace in which it must burn is a threefold one.

Who are the Three with whom the pupil must unite? Shankara explains them as Father, Mother and Guru, which, as we shall see, cleverly hides the actual inner meaning. Again we are reminded of the cryptic words in Light on the Path—"Regard the three truths. They are equal." The Three are in truth the three moments of the triple human monad, known in theosophical teachings as *Ātmā-Buddhi-Manas*. Hence Shankara's veiled words, for *Ātmā* is the male and generative Light of *Purusha*, *Buddhi*, a correlate on the human scale of *Mūlprakriti*, the great Mother, and *Manasa* the higher mind, is the *Āchārya* or Teacher.

We have up till now spoken of the higher *Manas* as if it in itself were the true higher self of man. This, however, is not so for, in itself, *Manas* is but the focus produced by the interaction of the two higher principles. It is a microcosm, corresponding on the purely human scale to the *Mahat* or Brāhmik Egg of the Cosmic scale, and, like the latter, is the Divine Son of the two Divine Parents. In actual fact, when we speak of the higher Self we refer, not to *Manas* alone, but to *Manas* as a focal centre through which shines forth the Light of the two higher. The true human I, Ego or Higher Self, is thus in reality a triple unity which derives its

title of monad from the fact that it is through a Point
"smaller than a mustard seed," as the Upanishad puts
it[1], that the triad manifests. It is the point-like window
through which the All looks out upon the All. Elsewhere I have termed it the Point of View.[2]

He who kindles successfully the Nachiketas Fire
unites his being with this Triple Monad. As for the
Three Acts, they are the three essential actions of the
Path, the acts of sacrifice, charity and self-discipline,
that are mentioned in the Gita[3] as the purifiers of those
who tread the Path of Wisdom, acts which are on no
account to be abandoned as mere bondage-bringing
illusions. But the three Acts in themselves are not
sufficient. In addition to them there must be the element
of Knowledge. Actions are useful, and, as the Gita
says, it is impossible to live without them. We should
therefore perform right action, the actions which help
along the Path. But even they in themselves will not
take us to the Goal. They must be backed by the knowledge of their inner significance. Hence the text tells
us that we must know and thoroughly realise by uniting
our being with that Shining Power, the one great
Knower, the Light of Pure Consciousness or consciring,[4] the Light that is born from the ultimate Mystery
of Darkness and is the "Light that lighteth every
man that cometh into the world." This Light, the
one Principle to which we should assimilate ourselves
(the true meaning of worship), is what we shall find
referred to later in this Upanishad as the *Shānta* or peaceful *Ātman*. Naturally, by assimilating oneself to it,

---

[1] *Chhāndogya* 3-14.
[2] See the present writer's *Yoga of the Bhagavat Gita*.
[3] Gita 18. 5.
[4] A term coined by the well-known philosopher E. D. Faw-
cett to avoid the ambiguity and suggestion of mere passivity
lurking in the word consciousness.

one gains unending peace for it is in itself the Peace of
God.

We should note also that the eighteenth verse
stresses the fact, as do all esoteric writings, that the
attainment is one which is to be accomplished here and
now. The Irish mystic A. E. rightly warns us against
all teachings that postpone their results till after death,
and our text similarly stresses the fact that it is here and
now, while still living on this earth, that the bonds of
death are to be destroyed, the sorrowless garment of
immortality to be put on. Death as such changes nothing and he who has not gained his immortality while
still 'alive' will not achieve it by the mere act of dying.
The *Ātman* in itself is of course eternal. The Higher
Self, enduring as it does throughout the age-long Cosmic Day, may well be described as endless; but the personal self, which is what we mean by our self in ordinary
speech, is neither immortal nor unending. It commenced at birth as the *Kārmic* inheritor of a previous personality, and though it will survive the event of physical death, perhaps for many centuries or even millennia,
it will not endure for ever. Nor will *it* be born again,
for its destiny is to be absorbed in the Father who sent
it forth and who will, in due time, send forth another
who shall be heir to its *Karma* as it was to that of its
predecessor. He who seeks to become immortal must
himself here and now become his Higher Self. There
is no other way. We now arrive at the third boon and
Nachiketas speaks again:

(20) *There is this doubt about a man who has gone Beyond, some saying that he exists, others that he exists no more.
This I desire to know as thy disciple (literally, being taught by
thee). This the third of my boons.*

The meaning of this boon has been missed by

almost all translators and commentators. The word
which has here been rendered 'gone Beyond' is *prete*,
which "Shankara" bluntly says means *mrite*—dead—and
in this reading nearly every one has followed him. But
such a rendering of the word makes no sense in the present context. In the first place, even before setting out
on his journey, Nachiketas, as we have seen, shows
that he is perfectly aware that as corn mortals ripen
and as corn they are born again. In other words, he
knows that after death man does not perish, but is born
again. Since then he has visited the very Halls of Death,
and still survives and, moreover, the very nature of his
second request shows that he is quite clear that after death
man goes—or at least can go—to bliss in the Heaven
World. Surely if any question of mere survival were
what is involved, the whole question about the Sacred
Fire would have been postponed till that were first
answered. To translate *prete* as 'died' is to make nonsense of the whole structure of the Upanishad.

Actually, the question is not one about survival
at all but about what happens to the individual Soul
after the attainment of liberation (*mukti*), a fact which
has once more been appreciated correctly by Madhva.[1]
The question is the very one that was asked of the Buddha more than once, whether, in Buddhist terms, the Arhat can be said to exist after Nirvāṇa, a question which
the Buddha always refused to answer, saying that to
affirm that he continued to exist would give rise to one
misunderstanding while to deny it would give rise to
others.

" Profound, measureless, unfathomable is He who
has found the Truth (the *Arhat,* he who has attained

[1] He equates *prete* with *mukte* : see his commentary on this Upanishad translated by Rai Bahadur Sirish Chandra Vidyāmana in
Sacred Books of the Hindus.

Nirvāṇa), profound even as the mighty ocean; the term reborn does not apply to him nor not reborn nor any combination of such terms. Everything by which the Truth-finder might be denoted has passed away for him utterly and for ever."[1]

It is this problem that Nachiketas is asking about (later as we shall see he terms it the Great Passing On)—truly a question to which some answer that 'he is' and some that 'he is not'! When a man attains to the final Goal, when he dies for the last time, liberated from all the bonds that bring ordinary men again and again to birth, what happens to him in that utter-passing away that takes place then, the Passing away that has been variously known as *Mukti, Moksha, Kaivalya* and *Nirvāṇa*. Nor was it only the teachings of the Buddha that gave rise to this doubt and speculation. In the *Brihadāranyaka Upanishad*, we find the great Seer Yājña-valkya explaining the mystery of the final state to his wife Maitreyi under particularly solemn circumstances.

"As a lump of salt dropped into water would dissolve and no one be able to pick it forth again, but wherever one should attempt to take it from would taste of salt—so truly this Great Being, endless and limitless, is one mass of Consciousness. (The separate self) comes out from these elements and into them it vanishes. Having *passed beyond* (*pretya*) there is no more separate consciousness (*sanjñā*). This is what I say."

Notice that in this passage the word *pretya* is used corresponding to the *prete* of the *Katha* and the meaning is the same. The word rendered consciousness (*sanjñā*) is also a technical term meaning a designation, the particular distinguishing sign of anything, hence a concept or clear notion. Hence also with the ambiguity which we have already referred to as inherent

----

[1] *Majjhima Nikaya*, Sutta 72.

in the word, clear, limited or particular consciousness, mind. It corresponds also to the term Name as used in the compound *Nāma-rūpa*, Name and Form, and denotes in reality the separate mental being, the Ego.

The *Bṛhadāranyaka* goes on :

"Maitreyi (his wife) said: by saying that there is no separate consciousness after the Passing On, you, O Lord, have bewildered me. Yajñavalkya replied—I am not saying anything bewildering. What I have said is sufficient for Knowledge."

He goes on to explain that where there is duality, there one has separate consciousness, one sees, hears, or thinks of another. "But where everything has become the One Self, whom and by what should one see, hear or think. Through what one should become conscious of that by which there is consciousness of the All. Whereby should one know the universal Knower."[1]

In the above passage, we have a clear reference to the same great problem, the same word used for the Passing On into liberation and the same doubt as to the meaning of the teaching. When a man is liberated from all the limitations of name and form, when he has ceased to identify himself with any one particular person or individual self, when he has become one with the All, how shall we say of him that he exists or does not exist ? Existence means a standing forth as something separate, a dualism between self and not-self—this and not-this. When the consciousness ceases to identify itself with any one point in the All more than with any other there is, in the strict sense of the term, no meaning in describing any particular being as existent. As far as strict

[1] *Bṛhadāranyaka Upanishad* 2. 4. 12-14. I am indebted to my friend Pandit Jagadish Chandra Chatterji for having pointed out the connection of this passage with the one in the *Kaṭha*.

logic is concerned that is correct but there is more than mere logic in words and the word existence signifies also something that we will term—if only to denote it—real being. Real being does not cease because standing forth (existence) ceases and therefore to say that he who is liberated has ceased to exist would be equally if not more misleading.

This ultimate state of those who are liberated, and not any question about mere survival after death, is the topic of Nachiketas' third boon; and it is interesting to note that when the early European Sanskritists first came upon the teaching about *Nirvāṇa*, a teaching that was for most of them something more or less entirely new, the very same controversy broke out among them, though on a purely intellectual plane, as to whether he who attains *Nirvāṇa* is annihilated or whether he enters into some incomprehensible state of being. Like the disputants mentioned in the text the scholars were divided, some saying that he exists, others that he exists no more.

Yama replies:

(21) *Even by the very Gods has (the answer to) this been doubted in former times. Nor is this very subtle subject one that is easy to understand, O Nachiketas. Choose another boon, do not, O do not press me. Release me from this promise.*

Nachiketas:

(22) *By the Gods indeed was this matter doubted and thou too, O Death, tellest me that it is not easy to understand. Another Teacher like thyself is not to be found, nor is there any other boon that is equal to this.*

Yama:

(23) *Choose sons and grandsons who shall live a hun-* ·

dred years; choose many cattle, elephants, horses and gold; choose broad lands to dwell in and for thyself to live as many autumns as thou wishest:

(24) If thou thinkest of any boon that is equal to this then choose it; wealth or longevity: be (ruler) of the great earth; I will make you an enjoyer of all desires.

(25) Whatever desires are difficult of attainment in this mortal world; ask for all desires at thy will. See these desirable maidens, seated on chariots and with instruments of music—their like cannot be had by man—by them, as my gift, be waited on and served; O Nachiketas, do not ask about (the Great) Dying.

Nachiketas replies:

(26) O Ender of all things; transient, ephemeral are all these. Moreover, they wear out the brightness of such sense powers as a mortal has. Even aeonic life is short (in comparison with that eternal state about which I have asked). Keep for thyself the chariots: thine be the song and dance.

(27) Not with wealth is man to be satisfied and if we should desire it, having once seen Thee (face to face) we shall surely obtain it. (As for life), so long as Thou rulest, so long shall we surely live. That (Knowledge) alone is the boon to be chosen by me.

(28) Having approached the Undecaying Immortal Ones, knowing (their unchanging nature) and reflecting analytically on the pleasures of lust and beauty, who is there among ageing mortals here below who would delight in long living (under such conditions as rule here)......Tell me, O Death, of that Great Passing On, concerning which people have such doubts. That which is wrapped in such great mystery (literally, that has entered into secrecy), that and no other boon shall Nachiketas ask.

It is unnecessary to say very much about these verses. We may point out how unintelligible they would be if the question was really one about personal survival. The Gods, Dwellers in the Heaven World, how should they have any doubts as to whether after death mortals came to them or not ? If, on the other hand, the question is taken as one about Ultimate Liberation the doubts of the Gods became quite intelligible since they, as Cosmic Powers, could not be certain about the nature of a state of Being that transcends the manifested universe altogether.[1] Only on this view, also, does Yama's extreme reluctance to speak have any meaning. Surely he need have no hesitation in speaking about what happens to man after death. Hence in verse 25 *Maraṇam* (literally dying) has been translated as the Great Dying in keeping with the Great Passing On (*Mahati Sāmparāye*) of verse 29 which Madhva states means the Great Blessing, i.e., Liberation.

Yama offers his pupil anything on earth rather than the knowledge of that ultimate state, but Nachiketas is firm and rejects all the proffered enjoyments. Notice how in verse 27 he shows his realisation that, so long as Yama shall endure, i.e., throughout the Cosmic Period, so long shall we continue to live. For Yama is the Higher Self and in him we are rooted. Not only that. He who has come face to face with the Higher Self and has become, as it were, that Self's disciple will never, should he need it, lack wealth. The state of our pockets as well as the state of our health is governed by the intentions of that Higher Self who is in fact the dispenser of *Karma*—subject of course to the all-ruling Cosmic Order in which he himself has his being. We think of the outer world of sense and of its various happenings as something separate from the inner worlds. But it is not so. As a bubble depends upon man's

---

[1] cf. *Gītā* X. 2 where Sri Krishna says: "The host of Gods know not my forthcoming."

breath, as ash depends upon fire, as a poem depends upon the poet's heart, so does this outer world depend upon and hang from the inner. Not by mere chance does anything whatever happen in this world. The 'bad luck' which pursues some men, so that nothing they undertake ever prospers, but is always wrecked by unforeseen accidents, that bad luck is but the displeasure of their own Higher Selves, which like Thompson's *Hound of Heaven*, bring it about that "all things betray Thee who betrayest Me." Conversely he who serves his Higher Self as a true disciple, listening for its lightest word and faithfully carrying it out, will never lack whatever means are necessary. Nachiketas' statement only echoes the words of Sri Krishna in the *Gītā*:—"To those who serve Me (the Higher Self) alone, thinking of no other, to those, ever united (to me), I bring all that they need."[1] Note again how in verse 28 Nachiketas is entirely aware that the Undecaying Immortal Ones exist and that he himself has approached them. He who has once seen their calm immortal eyes can care no more for any life but theirs. He knows moreover that with the help of the sacred Fire he can attain to that undecaying life. How should he care for the transient pleasures of men. Therefore he refuses all other offers. He will know of the Great, the Ultimate Mystery of which it has been written:—

"Hold fast to that which has neither substance nor existence......Look only on that which is invisible alike to the inner and the outer sense."[2]

This is the Knowledge that Nachiketas seeks. With no other will he be content for there alone is the ultimate Knowledge, the *Paramārthik* Truth. All else is relative knowledge, true as far as it goes: this alone

[1] *Gītā* IX. 22.
[2] *Light on the Path.*

48

is that Knowledge which, being known, all is known, the Knowledge of that Reality whose being is so incomprehensible to us that the great Buddhist teachers could find no better word to denote it than *Shūnya*, the "Void," while the Vedantins designated it simply as 'That'.

CHAPTER II

Nachiketas having shown his determination to attain the ultimate Knowledge, having refused to be tempted aside from his path by the lure of desires, the Initiator proceeds to impart the teaching which will enable his pupil to find in and for himself the answer to his question. Once more we may quote from *Light on the Path*:—

"Inquire of the earth, the air, the water, of the secrets they hold for you.

The development of your inner senses will enable you to do this."

In the terms of our Upanishad we may say that the three elements, 'Earth,' 'Air,' and 'Water' have given birth to the sacred Nachiketas Fire, the means to the knowledge of the secrets of nature. ,

"Inquire of the Holy Ones of the earth of the secrets they hold for you.

The conquering of the desires of the outer senses will give you the right to this."

This stage too has been passed; for the pupil has successfully resisted all the blandishments of desire and that, too, not by the mere asceticism of the will which forcibly tramples them under foot, but by the surer light of discriminative knowledge before which they fall in lifeless disintegration. Resolutely has he adhered to his determination and confidently has he approached the Holy One, the One Initiator, the Higher Self than whom, as he declares in verse 22, no better Teacher is to be found. From that Higher Self comes all the teaching which follows and, as we read again in

Chapter II

Light on the Path:

"Inquire of the inmost the One, of its final secret, which it holds for you through the ages.

The great and difficult victory, the conquering of the desires of the individual soul is a work of ages: therefore expect not to obtain its reward until ages of experience have been accumulated."

Insight into the futility of all personal desires is one thing. Their utter eradication and uprooting from the heart is another. This is the great task which the teaching is to accomplish, leaving at its conclusion the pupil standing on the verge of the ultimate mystery which none can impart, the wings of the soul strengthened and purified in preparation for the last great flight, "the flight of the Alone to the Alone."

The teaching therefore commences with the need for renunciation of all personal or individual desire.

(1) *The better is one thing: other indeed is that which is more pleasant. Both these attach the Purusha, (the pure Light), but to different objects (namely liberation and bondage). Of them well-being comes to him who chooses the better, while he who chooses the more pleasant fails to attain the Goal.*

(2) *The better and the more pleasant both approach man. Having examined them from all sides, the wise man discriminates between them. He chooses the better rather than the more pleasant, while the foolish, through desire to have and hold (objects of desire), chooses the more pleasant.*

(3) *Thou indeed, O Nachiketas, having meditated on the nature of pleasant, and of pleasant-seeming desires, hast cast them from thee. Not by thee were accepted those golden chains laden by which so many men sink down.*

At the very outset of the Path, we are faced with the necessity of having to discriminate between the

51

two voices which whisper perpetually in our hearts, the voice of duty and the voice of desire. Man as the central point, the pivot of the Universe, stands between two worlds, the upper and harmonious world of the *Buddhi,* and the lower and discordant world of desire. The latter, it is true, is a reflection of the former—*demon est deus inversus*—but the inversion in question is a very important one. Above, all is harmony, peace and the divine unity in which

> "All things by a law divine
> In one another's being mingle."

Below is the world of separation, of strife and of discord. Both are reflected in the mirror of the heart.

The Gita, too, urges the disciple to set aside the promptings of attraction and repulsion, the positive and negative aspects of the desire principle and to guide his actions by the voice of *Swadharma,* or duty, which corresponds to what is here termed *Shreya,* the better or more excellent. It is often said now-a-days that what is sometimes called conscience is nothing but the voice of racial, social, and, above all, parental approval, and it is certainly true that much that passes for the voice of conscience is little, if anything, more than that. When we have admitted this, however, we have said nothing more than that, in the ordinary man, the voice of conscience, like other things in his psyche, is overlaid with baser matter. In exactly the same way the perception of beauty in art or nature is overlaid with racial and social conventions, to the great prejudice of the pure aesthetic judgment. How many there are who admire a certain picture just because it is considered to be by a great master and who frequent concerts for no better reason than that it is considered cultured to care for classical music.

Chapter II

The voice of conscience is in a very similar position to the voice of beauty, the so-called aesthetic faculty, and in point of fact the two are by no means altogether separate for both are in reality perceptions of the element of harmony that is derived from the harmony of the *buddhi,* one being concerned particularly with one aspect, the other with another. Truth, Beauty and Goodness are the three sides of a triangle, the triangle of the three-faced *buddhi,* and no one of them can stand alone.

Of course, it is true that in ordinary men those perceptions of value are tangled up and alloyed with much base metal. Hence it is that the spiritual alchemist has first of all to purify the elements with which he is dealing, to separate out, as the old symbolism phrased it, the Sulphur, Salt and Mercury, which together compose the body of all things, including of course the body of the human psyche. Just as the artist learns to appraise, with more and more precision, the purely aesthetic qualities of an object, so must the disciple of this path learn to discriminate more and more accurately those qualities of an action which, for want of a better term, we must call ethical.

To put it briefly, an action is 'good' or 'better' just in proportion as it manifests the harmony of the *buddhi,* the unity of life, and the interconnectedness of all things. It is 'bad' in proportion as, ignoring that underlying unity, it is designed exclusively for the benefit of a separate centre, the personal self of the doer.

It is this that the principle of desire is always luring us to do. As the Upanishad says, out of desire to have and hold objects for oneself, the ordinary man is always choosing the more pleasant course, the one which seems most gratifying to him personally. The wise man, on the other hand, carefully examines the

53

proposed action from all sides and acts in the way most in accord with the principle of harmony. But is it not difficult in practice to disentangle these two voices? Of course it is: never has it been said that this Path is an easy one. No true disciple will be put off by the difficulties in the Path. All he requires to know is that this is what has to be done: quickly or slowly he will do it. As he proceeds with his work of self-purification the process will become easier, but, even at the outset, when faced by two alternative ways of action, it is usually possible, *if one really wishes to*, to see which of them appeals more to that in one which is recognisably one's better self. At first, owing to the impure state of our psyches, we shall have to be content with a relative purity of motive, with the 'better,' often in the sense of the lesser of two evils; but that is only the beginning and with every decision the psychic elements will assume greater purity, so that it will daily become more and more clear which is the *Shreya*, the more excellent, and which the merely *preya*, the more pleasant.

It may, however, not be out of place to mention that there are, as on all unfrequented ways, dangers on this Path. It is the Path of knowledge and gradually he who follows it will come to realise that much, very much, of what he considered right or wrong in the past is only such by social convention. So far he has been supported by external props, the 'thou shalt' and 'thou shalt not' of external morality. One by one the artificial nature |of| these props will be seen by him and one by one they will fall away from him. He has to learn to stand in his own strength alone, supported only by his own inner perception of what is in accordance with the cosmic harmony. It is just at this point that dangers assail him. If his development is unbalanced, if his intellect has outrun the perception of his soul, those props are sure to fall away before he is ready to stand firmly on his own inner feet, for "even ignorance is better than Head-learning with no Soul-wisdom to guide it"[1] and "before the Soul can stand in the presence of the Masters its feet must be washed in the blood of the heart."[2]

Only too often does it happen that 'head-learning' cuts away the traditional outer sanctions before there is sufficient 'Soul wisdom' to perceive the true and inner ones. Then the pupil becomes a law unto himself, one who can see no sanctions anywhere save those of his own egoistic desires; for the mind, however brilliantly it may seem to shine in its own light, is, when not the willing servant of the *buddhi*, the forced bondslave of the underlying tides of desire. The antinomianism which has so often made its appearance in mystical societies and brotherhoods affords clear proof of the truth of this statement. Desire, though slain by us, is only too frequently able to rise once more from the dead to work our destruction.

Just as Arjuna had to slay his former Gurus in the battle of Kurukshetra, so the old props must go, in order that the sapling which is to grow into the great Tree[3] may learn to stand free and untrammelled. Sorrowful indeed is the lot of the many, shut in on all sides by the ignorance of externality. But far more unfortunate is the lot of those who, as the *Ishopanishad* has it, are devoted to head-learning (*Vidyā*) alone and whose props are cut away before they have learned to stand. They fall "into an even greater darkness," a darkness out of which it is far harder to emerge, the darkness of an intellectually enlightened selfishness.

---

[1] *Voice of the Silence.*
[2] *Light on the Path.*
[3] In some old symbolisms initiates were known as Trees, the Cedars of Lebanon.

This is a topic that is treated more explicitly in the
Iṣhopaniṣhad. Here too, however, it is referred to in
the first verse of this section which states that both of
these paths, the path of the excellent and the path of the
pleasant, bind or attach the pure Light of Consciousness or *Purusha.* We may remember also the statement of the Gita that the stainless and harmonious
guṇa of *sattva* also binds by causing the soul to become
attached to its inner bliss, the bliss of harmony and
knowledge.[1]

Increase of the harmonious or *sāttvik* element
of the psyche leads to an increase of peace and knowledge, but even this is an attachment, a bondage for
the pure Light of the Atman, for all peace that is not
the ultimate 'Peace of God' is transient and all knowledge
that is not the transcendent and ineffable Knowledge
of the Brahman is but relative. The wise man, however, makes use of the relative light and harmonious *Sattva*, the Path of the Excellent, as a raft
with which to float over the dark and stormy waters
of desire. Having reached to the Other Side, the
raft too must be abandoned, since to retain it then would
be a further bondage.

Before passing on we may note that Nachiketas
is not one who has accepted the golden chains of
desire which sink so many souls beneath the waters.
Again and again we see the golden promise and
soaring idealism of youth gradually compromising
with use and wont, gradually learning, little by little,
to accept the claims of the expedient, if only temporarily
for the present, instead of the claims of the Right.
Gradually the Pleasant, success as the world counts
success, comes in answer to their call but as it comes
it loads their neck with its golden chains and they sink

[1] Gita 14. 6.

beneath the weight. The dead gold of matter drives out the bright and living Gold of the Sun, so that, leaving the latter's bright Path, they gradually descend by the reversed alchemy of desire, through the brazen complacency of middle age, to a leaden and unlovely death.

Such is the path of Desire, a path trodden by those who listen to the voice of the Pleasant. He who would tread successfully the other Path must learn from the very outset to shun even the slightest and most insidious whispers of that voice. As a thin thread, subtler than spider's gossamer, it enters the soul: as a great python, thicker than a man's body, will it crush out that soul's life if allowed to remain. As when we walk along an unfrequented jungle path, we feel the touch of thin fine threads upon our faces, so as we journey through the dark forests of the world, the subtle threads of Desire make contact with our hearts. If we brush them off at once, all is well; but if we let them remain, if we give them time to adhere and enter in, it is not long before, like the air-borne rootlets of some tropical parasites, they grow into an enveloping network which slowly drains the heart-tree of all its life, leaving behind a hollow ruin which will fall at the first breath of winter winds.

As a thread too comes to us the other, the higher Voice, but it is the life-saving thread which is shot out by rocket to the sinking vessel, the thread which will serve to draw over in succession a twine, a cord, a rope and finally a hawser, along which all the crew can pass to safety. He who entertains and makes fast *this* thread, will in the end stand safely on the Land beyond the waves.

(4) *Far apart, contradictory and leading to different ends are this pair, Ignorance and what is known as Know-*

ledge. Nachiketas I consider to be a seeker after Knowledge, since the multitude of desires could not move or tear thee away.

(5) Revolving in the midst of Ignorance, wise in their own conceit, considering themselves learned, wandering hither and thither, the fools go round and round like blind men led by the blind.

It is perhaps hardly necessary to say that the terms Ignorance and Knowledge, *Avidyā* and *Vidyā*, as used in Upanishadic Texts do not refer to ordinary worldly ignorance and knowledge. Neither on the other hand, is it correct to take, as is done by some, *Vidyā* as meaning a purely metaphysical knowledge, knowledge, in fact, of the subtleties of some particular system of 'Indian philosophy.' *Vidyā* and *Avidyā* are in reality two ways of what in the most general sense we must term knowing, two ways of being aware of or consciring the cosmos. There is only one universal reality, the universe with which we are concerned, but that universe, or even this world, to limit the discussion still farther, is very much more extensive than is believed by scientists and men in general. The one world is capable of being perceived (conscired) in many distinct ways of which we may distinguish seven main ones.

There is or used to be a children's toy which consisted of a picture or black and white drawing which if looked at from one point of view, was of one subject, say a cottage in the midst of a wood, and if looked at from a different angle, revealed a quite different scene, say someone cooking his dinner over a fire. Neither of these representations existed in themselves so to speak; both were special points of view of a single matrix of lines and dots.

Somewhat in the same way, the seven modes of

consciousness, to which we have referred, give rise to seven distinct world-experiences which are what we term the seven planes or levels of experience, each seeming quite distinct but each being in reality a separate reading of the one psychic matrix which is the world or universe as a whole. We are not here concerned with the description of these seven planes but with the general idea that the world is a psychic matrix which some see in one way, others in another. Some, that is, pick out from it one type of pattern, others another: "The fool sees not the same tree as the wise man sees." In a very general way, all men in their waking consciousness are aware of perceiving the same, or what they believe to be the same world. This, however, is because of the modal similarity of ordinary waking consciousness all the world over and is no evidence whatever of an ordinary common-sense world existing independently in its own right.

We are here concerned with two great ways of consciring or being aware of the world. One stresses the harmony and interconnectedness of all the elements which make up that world while the other stresses their separateness, mutual independence and consequent strife. The first of these modes of experience may be described as the mode of unity, the second as that of diversity. In the first, everything is seen as part of a whole, as connected with a whole and as harmonious in that whole: in the second as separate, as independent and as struggling for its own place in the sunlight. The position was very neatly expressed by an old Sufi, that the present writer once met in Lucknow, who said: "that which makes one out of two is truth; that which makes two out of one is falsehood."

It is these two ways of *seeing* or experiencing the world which are termed by the Upanishadic writers

Vidyā and *Avidyā*, Knowledge and Ignorance. Referring them to the seven already mentioned, we may say that Knowledge consists, roughly speaking, of the three higher ways of perceiving, in other words, of the three higher planes, while Ignorance consists of the three lower ones. The pure *manas*, or individual Ego, is the central point between the two, the pivot of the whole, and one which takes its colouring from what it sees, becoming thus Higher Self, or *buddhi-manas* or lower self *kāma-manas*. The former sees in the mode of Knowledge, the latter in the mode of Ignorance.

Note, however, that these modes are further divisible. Hence our text speaks not of Knowledge but only of *what is known* as such, since the ultimate Knowledge, the completely unitive seeing, takes us beyond the dualism of manifestation into the non-dualism of the unitive experience, in which seer and seeing and seen are no longer separate or separable. "Our way then takes us beyond knowing; there may be no wandering from unity; knowing and knowable must all be left aside. Every object of thought even the highest we must pass by for all that is good is later than this......No doubt we should not speak of seeing; but we cannot help talking in dualities, seen and seer, instead of boldly, the achievement of unity. In this seeing we neither hold an object nor trace distinction; there is no two. The man is changed, no longer himself nor self belonging; he is merged with the supreme, sunken into it, one with it......only in separation is there duality. This is why the vision baffles telling; we cannot detach the supreme to state it; if we have seen something thus detached we have failed of the supreme."[1]

[1] Plotinus vi. 9. 4 and 10.

Chapter II

It is for this reason, that the text speaks only of what is known as *Vidyā*, of relative Knowledge, as we might express it now-a-days. Such *Vidyā* is one of the pair of opposites that make up the whole texture of the manifested universe; the true Knowledge is beyond all manifestation and is complete in itself.

The majority of men care not for the Knowledge. In the name of commonsense and of practicality, they prefer to perceive the differences between things. They see a stone or plant as just a stone or plant, as something complete and standing in its own being, instead of seeing it as it really is—a focus in the network of relationships that make up the cosmos. It is true that modern physics has advanced somewhat on the road which leads to the perception of the unity of all things, and isolated sentences of great truth can be gleaned from the works of certain scientific writers. But the enlightenment attained is a purely intellectual one. Their real vision, as shown by their everyday thoughts, remains on the plane of separation and therefore of the Ignorance. When we leave the field of science and turn to that of everyday life, a similar situation is revealed. The ordinary man spends his entire life in the pursuit of objects of desire. Such pursuit is the very quintessential Ignorance, for it is based on a lack of knowledge of the true nature both of the self which desires and of the objects desired.

These objects are not things in themselves which can be acquired. Rather they are so many ways of seeing what is ever present.

"Desire possessions above all."

"But those possessions must belong to the pure soul only and be possessed therefore by all pure souls equally, and thus be a special property of the whole only when united."[1]

The Self, as we have seen, is the window through which the All looks out upon the All. It is thus the centre of a net-work of relationships that extend throughout the whole universe. To have the true possessions that are referred to in the above passage, the individual Ego and its reflection, the personal self, must attain to consciousness of all these threads of relationship. As long as it sees itself as something isolated and objects of desire as isolated things which it can acquire, so long is it dwelling in the midst of the Ignorance running hither and thither after what is essentially an illusion. However learned it may be in the mode known as science (*Vidyā*), it is really caught in the net of nescience; itself blind to the truth, it follows teachers who, if possible, are blinder still. Thus as Christ said, both fall into the Pit, a saying whose full implications are only understood when it is realised that to occultism this world is known as the Pit or hell into which the souls are thrown down. We may remember also that, to the Orphic initiates, the physical body was the Tomb in which is buried the living Soul.

In proportion, on the other hand, as the individual self becomes conscious of its relatedness to all things, to that extent it enters the realm of the Knowledge and, in acquiring knowledge of its relatedness, acquires possessions in the only true and real sense in which they can be acquired. In such a case, knowledge of an existing fact, that of relatedness, replaces the striving after illusory objects considered as separate. Hence as the soul leaves the realms of Ignorance and enters those of Knowledge, the burning thirst of desire will cease. Instead of trying desperately and vainly to

[1] *Light on the Path.*

acquire increase of stature, enhanced fullness of being, by impossible additions from without, the soul will bend its efforts towards realising the stature, the fullness of being, that it already and inherently possesses within itself. Therefore it has been said "mingle your being in that of all around you" and therefore, also, the sign that a man is ready to tread the Path of Knowledge is that the waves of desire should be subsiding in his heart. So long as these waves surge and riot in his being, so long is he attached to the Ignorance, and, interested though he may be in some of the many phases of the hidden Teachings, such interest will in reality be a self-centred one, a desire for personal attainments of some sort. To such a one the true Teacher will not and indeed cannot respond. This is a topic to which we shall have to recur in connection with the later verses of this section. Here we shall only point out that it is because the multitude of desires are unable to tear and rend the unity of Nachiketas' heart, that the Teacher recognises in him a true aspirant for the Hidden Wisdom, a candidate for initiation in the Sacred Knowledge.

(6) *The Passing On is never clear to the fool, to him who like a child acts carelessly, befooled by the delusion of possessions. He who thinks that this world alone exists and that there is no other, again and again comes under my control.*

Here we have the plain statement of the matter. He who believes that possessions can be acquired and consequently strives after them is, however learned in the wisdom of this world, a mere undeveloped child with regard to the hidden Wisdom. The true nature of the Great Passing On into ultimate Being can in no way become manifest to him, for he is still looking for it where it does not exist, namely, in a vision that is based on the idea of separateness. However great the Teacher and however true the Teaching that is set before him, it would become a falsity in his mind, for he would apprehend it only in terms of his own ignorant vision of the nature of things. He who thinks, for instance, that this world alone exists, that physical existence is the only type of being, is bound to go utterly astray when he hears of the Teaching. If told that man continues to exist after physical death, he will inevitably conceive that existence in terms of what he now considers such. Hence will arise such foolish doctrines as that of the resurrection of the body, though in truth even this doctrine has a profound inner meaning and has only become a thing of folly because of its misapprehension by just such 'children' as our text refers to.

Not even the nature of ordinary after-death experience can be grasped by him who sees and believes only in this world. Whatever view he may hold and set forth concerning that state is inevitably bound to be either meaningless or else untrue. He who literally believes in no other world will of course hold no view at all. At least he should not, though in point of fact he usually does, for he holds the view of annihilation, that which the Buddhists referred to as *ucchedavāda*. But we must cast our net wider than this and include in its sweep, not only those who say they do not believe, but also those who have what is known in exoteric religion as belief, and who are in consequence what the Buddha, again, called *shāshwata-vādis* or perpetualists, holding that the self persists unchanged and forever.

What is ordinarily known as belief is doubtless a stage higher than the negativism of sheer unbelief (which, by the way, always dogs it like a shadow), but to be a believer, as the word is usually used, by

no means provides the key to knowledge. Not belief, in the sense of willed affirmation, but *seeing* is
what is required though it is true that, at the beginning,
that seeing will be done by the Higher Self and will
only filter down to the personality in the form of what
we have already described as true Faith, the Faith that
is a veiled form of actual perception. In truth we may
paraphrase the words of the Upanishad thus:—

"He who sees (whatever he may 'believe') this
physical universe as the only reality can never understand what is beyond it. To understand the beyond,
even the beyond-death, let alone that Great Beyond,
which is the subject of the teaching, it is essential that
the disciple should be able to *see* other aspects of the
universe, if only with the eye of true Faith, and that
he should see them here and now in ordinary work-a-
day life. Only then will he be able to commence that
transmutation of the lower self, that polishing of the
heart's mirror which will enable it to reflect the starry
constellations of eternal truth that shine above him
in the heavens of the *Buddhi*. In those Stars are all
Knowledge, all that has happened in the past, all that
happens now and all that will ever happen, is written
in their golden letters of light; not in the sense of the
crude fatalism that is one of the illusions of the Ignorance, but in the sense that they stand outside our time
in the upper world of Light, while their apparent or
relative motion is reflected as the changing events below."[1]

The disciple can be quite sure that if those Stars

[1] The reader may ask in what way this differs from fatalism.
The answer he must find out for himself, for it cannot be expressed
in words except in so far as we can say that determinism and in-
determinism are two of the opposites and therefore neither in itself is true. We may also add that the 'Stars' referred to both are
and are not the familiar heavenly bodies.

are not reflected in the mirror of his heart, it is because
it is covered with the dust of desire. Let him clean
and polish it carefully and he will begin to see the so-
called other worlds, the non-physical aspects of the
universe, first in the relatively dim mode of Faith and
later with the clarity of open-eyed vision.

Man is a citizen of three worlds, in all of which
even now he has his being. As long as he sees and
knows only the physical universe, so long do the other
worlds, dark and unperceived by him, exert upon him
their relentless, fatal pull. Fate is a very real aspect
of our lives as long as we remain in the Ignorance,
as real as the other aspect of freedom. What we
call fate is the pulling and moulding of our lives from
sources of which we are unconscious. Where there
is the Light of consciousness all is freedom; wherever
to us that Light does not penetrate is Fate. To the
adept *siddha* whose consciousness enfolds the whole
range of manifested being there is no fate at all, while
to the stone whose consciousness is all but entirely
shut in there is little else.[1] The Path of Light is the
path of mastery. Those whose vision is limited to the
physical and especially those (and they are not a few)
who deliberately limit their vision in order that no considerations of other worlds may limit or check their sensual
enjoyments, pay the price of such limitation in an
inevitable subjection to the unperceived, in other
words to Fate. As Yama says, 'again and again they
come under my control.' They who seek unlimited
freedom for their personal desires are caught in the
toils of a relentless fate. They who while living will
not in freedom die the mystic death, must in consequence

---

[1] Even in the ultimate realms of physical matter, there is, as
modern physics confirms, an element of freedom or indetermin-
ism.

bow to compulsion and tread not once but many times
the dark and gloomy path of ordinary death. Once
more we are reminded of the Mystery teaching already
quoted: "the greater Deaths do greater lots obtain."

Having set Nachiketas on the Path to Knowledge,
lest he should be discouraged by the apparent lack
of progress which afflicts so many pupils, Yama proceeds to set forth the extreme difficulty and the wonder
of the Knowledge, the necessity also for a competent
Guru or Teacher if further advance is to be made.

(7) *That State (the* Sāmparāye) *which the many do not
even hear of and which, even having heard of, many cannot
understand—wonderful is its Teacher, skilful its obtainer,
wonderful indeed is he who knows It, taught by an able Teacher.*

(8) *It is not to be understood properly when taught by
an inferior type of teacher, even if thought about in many ways;
(and yet) unless taught by another there is no path to it, for it
is unreachable by argument, being subtler even than the subtle
(literally the atomlike central point, the* Jīva *or Higher Self).*[1]

(9) *This wisdom*[2] *which thou hast attained is not to be*

[1] The grammatical construction of this verse is very ambi-
guous and many renderings exist, which those interested must
consult in more learned books than this one. Shankara himself gives four possible explanations. Possibly the ambiguity
is deliberate and more than one meaning is intended. For instance, *ananya prokite gatiratra nāsti*, here rendered as, unless taught
by another there is no path to it may also mean 'when taught by
one who is not separate from It', one who is rooted in It, or again,
alternatively by one who, not being separate from It (the Atman),
is thus not separate from the pupil's own Self, there is no doubt,
(in one version Shankara takes *gatih* in this sense), or, no further
transmigration in the worlds of birth and death. Ancient writers
frequently compressed many meanings into one sentence and it
is quite possible that either or both of these alternatives are also
included in the text.

[2] Taking *mati* as a synonym for *buddhi.*

gained by any process of logical thought (nor is it to be destroyed by such either).[1] *Yet when taught by another it is easy to be known. Thou, O dearest Nachiketas, art of true resolve. May we have such another questioner as thee.*

It is not possible to attain to the Wisdom by means of any process of logical thinking. For this there is a very good reason, since the process of logical thinking is essentially an analytic one. The mind picks out a single point in the complex of experience and traces from that point a network of relationships. Such relating of all experience to and from a single point is the very essence of the mind which is itself a single Point within the Whole. But the divine Knowledge is of a different nature. It is a synthetic Knowledge which we may symbolically refer to the circumference rather than the centre of a circle, a knowledge of things in their all-togetherness rather than in their separateness. In the mental mode, we start by isolating individual elements and proceed by inference, if at all, to the knowledge of the whole. In this other mode, which we may as well term the mode of the *buddhi*, the Whole is grasped in experience and the knowledge of the individual comes from the fact that that Whole is reflected in each separate point or lesser unity. Such Knowledge is thus related to the deductive knowledge of academic philosophy, but, while related, the two must not be confused; for deductive knowledge, as known in the scholastic world, is a matter of reasoning from certain principles, taken as established, from purely mental postulates; while the Knowledge with which we are here concerned, starts from nothing mental at all but from *experience*, and proceeds to *see* rather than to *think* the pattern of the Whole as it is reflected in the part. It

[1] Madhva holds that there is a play on words here.

is the famous third Knowledge of Spinoza which proceeds from Knowledge of the Whole to knowledge of the parts.

It will thus be seen that, when the Upanishad states that it is not to be attained by any logical reasoning, it is not, as sometimes supposed, merely vaguely praising the Knowledge by placing it out of reach of current modes of knowing, but is making a definite statement for a definite reason. As long as we confine ourselves to the purely mental mode we are condemned to chase our own tails for ever. Starting from a point, we may wander from point to point all over the surface of the heavenly sphere; in the end, to *that* very point we must come back. No matter with how fine a network of lines we try to cover and map out the sphere, we cannot do so, for the unity which is its most fundamental characteristic forever eludes this point-to-point mental mode.

As remarked in a footnote, Madhva considers that the word rendered as "attained" also means 'destroyed'. Just as the mental mode cannot achieve this Knowledge, so it cannot destroy it either. This is the reason for the serene confidence of the Seers in the face of hostile and destructive criticism. That which is not established by reasoning cannot by reasoning be overturned. At the most the mind may legitimately call in question the appropriateness of the verbal expression that is inevitably made use of in the attempt to communicate the truth. But only a fool will expect the sign-post to resemble the town to which it points the way, and only an academic will suppose that an inadequate expression affects the truth of the *experience* which it was sought to express. This is what has so seldom been understood about the six *darshanas*, the so-called systems of Indian philosophy. They are types of expression, each adapted to a particular type of mind, to which that form of expression will make the strongest and clearest appeal. The Experience that each seeks to express is one and the same, however differently it may be dressed in words. India has, no doubt, always had its sectarians, those who believed that their chosen system was uniquely true. But besides these there have always been others, and it is they who have most typified the genius of India, men who have realised the interdependence of all the systems and who, though they may have made special use of one, were always ready to restate their position in terms of any of the others.

"That which is known by Shaivas as Shiva, as Brahman by the Vedāntins, as Buddha by the Buddhists, as Arhat by the Jainas, and as all-ruling Karma by the Mimāmsakas. May that Hari, Lord of the Triple-world grant us the Fruit we desire."

Such expressions as this can be found throughout the Indian tradition, which from the far away Vedik times, has ever proclaimed that "the Real is One; (though) the learned call It by many names." Even now, though there are those who are willing to give their minds into sectarian keeping, the general spirit of India rejects such limitations and instinctively feels, ⋅ ⋅ ⋅ with the Emperor Ashoka, that to decry the religious teaching of another is to expose the weakness of one's own.

Our verse, from which we have wandered somewhat, goes on to emphasise the need of a Guru or Teacher. The Knowledge, to borrow a convenient modern phrase, is 'knowledge by acquaintance' not 'knowledge by description.' As such it is necessary that the disciple should be initiated into it by one who has already experienced it for only such a one can use words in such a way as to break through their surface reference and allow their underlying meaning to shine forth. Only such a one, in fact, can "speak with authority and not as the scribes." Such speech, unless we deliberately shut our hearts, we instinctively recognise. Deep in our hearts is that which knows its truth and even if the mind deliberately and out of egoism refuses its assent, it cannot carry with it the whole of the psyche. Deep within the normal layers of consciousness the truth is accepted and though the mind may protest and kick with all its might, it is safely tethered by the heel and it can never escape the inner acceptance. It may indeed refuse it a place in its consciousness, and, in its efforts to drown the voice, become a persecutor of the truth in others. Nevertheless it can never escape, and, in the end, there will be one of those sudden conversions that so bewilder the superficial and set them talking about supernatural intervention. It was *before* he started persecuting the Christians that Paul's soul gave itself to Christ. The dramatic incident on the road to Damascus was only the final and violent overpowering of his ego-mind. Incidentally such 'sudden conversions' are by no means entirely satisfactory. The violence used first by and then on the mind has, like all violence, to be paid for later, and those who are not committed to an orthodox view will find no difficulty in tracing certain unsatisfactory aspects of the Pauline Christian tradition to the original violence of his conversion.

Fundamentally the Guru is the Soul itself or to speak more exactly, the divine world of the *buddhi*, the noetic world of Plotinus, which is to be found in its entirety reflected in the hearts of each one of us. That divine Soul is spoken of as 'other' because it is the matrix out of which the individual 'I' emerges, the background or stage on which, like a performing ape, the mind goes through its tricks. It cannot be too emphatically stated that the Knowledge is in the Soul,

and of the Soul, and, truest of all, is itself that Soul.
Ashwaghosha contrasts the enlightenment that is gained
by effort with the enlightenment that existed all the time.
By the former is brought about nothing but a manifestation of the latter.[1]

Unfortunately, "having eyes we see not and
having ears we hear not." The voice of the *buddhi*,
the inner Guru, is sounding the whole time but our
ears are so deafened by the clashing of embattled desires that we are unable to hear it. Even if we 'believe'
in other worlds, we are apt to consider that practical
affairs are to be guided by considerations of this world
alone, and no voice has much chance of getting itself
heard unless it can manifest to us through our physical
sense of hearing.

It is for this reason that though exceptional men,
or, to speak more truly, men who have advanced far
on the Path in previous lives and are now but recapi-
tulating stages already achieved, appear sometimes to
have scaled the Peaks with the aid of the inner Guru
alone, the ordinary aspirant needs an embodied Teacher,
one who, though seeming 'other' than the disciple himself, can make manifest on this plane the voice of that
Self which is in truth the Self of all and has sometimes
accordingly been spoken of as *Vaishvānara*, the Universal-
in-all-men. To such a voice obedience, as always, must
be with the free-will of the disciple, for there can be no
coercion on the Path. Addressed as it is, however, to
our physical ears, it must at least be *heard*. It follows
that those (and they are many) who seek for a Guru
who will spirit them along the Path with a wave of the

[1] *Awakening of Faith in the Mahayana*: Susuki's translation
p. 62. Enlightenment *a priori* is contrasted with enlightenment
a posteriori. Though enlightenment *a posteriori* is gained no more
than enlightenment *a priori*.

hand are seeking for what does not and cannot exist. As one such Guru has said: "out of discussion we call to vision, to those desiring to see we point the path: our teaching is a guiding in the way; the seeing must be the very act of him who has made the choice."[1]

Almost indispensable as is the embodied Teacher and immensely advantageous as it is to have found that personal Guru through whom the impersonal Voice can speak to *us*, equally indispensable is it that the disciple should be ready to take advantage of the wonderful privilege which his previous and unaided efforts have entitled him to. How great a privilege it is is known to those who have been fortunate enough to find their Guru, for, though there are wonderful enough notions current among those who are only seeking for Him, the truth, as always, is far more wonderful than the fantastic fairy-tales which fill the public ear.

"Prostrations to that Guru who has unveiled for me that Unbroken Sphere which pervades this world of separate things."[2]

Sanskrit books are full of signs by which the true Guru can be recognised but such lists are of little use in practice. More to the point are the equivalent lists of the qualities which should be possessed by the disciple and these will repay careful study. Our present text mentions one and that a most essential one, truth of resolve.. The Guru is recognised in moments of calm and insight, in such moments as visit the disciple as peaks of inner harmony in which for the time being the

[1] Plotinus 6. 9. 4.
[2] Actually *charācharam* of moving and unmoving things. The Hymn to the Guru from which this verse is quoted is full of expressions of the sort that prompt Westerners to talk of "that most incomprehensible of Hindu idolatries, the idolatry of the Guru !" Such people do not realise who or what is the Guru who is referred to in such glorious terms.

distracting voices of desire are lulled to sleep. At such times he is able to hear with his inner ear and to recognise the voice that speaks to him from without as the true echo of the Voice within his heart. In the very nature of things, however, such moments of insight cannot and do not persist, and the disciple will need all his determination if in the intervening periods of darkness, a darkness that will seem blacker than ever by contrast with the light he has experienced, he is to continue to hold his course by the star he has glimpsed but of which he has now only a memory to guide him. Again and again at such moments he will be tempted to turn back to the shore lights he has left behind him, again and again he will be tempted to regret that he ever embarked upon this voyage. Once he has left the safety of the harbour in which so many spend their whole lives playing at the voyage, troubles and dangers of all sorts will assail him. The Star, which shone so clearly, becomes, as we have said, dimmed by clouds. From time to time cold banks of fog drift over him and the great waves of the deep which had been artificially stilled within the harbour breakwater, now rise in fury, threatening to engulf him and testing in every plank the sea-worthiness of his vessel.

It is here that all his "truth of resolve" will be needed and such resolve cannot be found among the eddying desires which make up the personal self. Only if he can draw on the will of the Higher Self, if he can feel himself gripped firmly in the strong hand of that inner determination, will it be possible for him to carry on. The truth is that the ordinary and lower self of the disciple is menaced with destruction and knows it. Hence its panic rage, a rage which only he who can firmly trust and identify himself with the Higher can hope at first to ride out and later to quell.

It may be asked and it is a point which is confusing

to many, who is the 'he' who is to do this and that, to unite with the higher, to quell the lower and so forth ? The answer is that there is no 'he' at all in the sense of an independent entity: still less is there a set of 'he's like Chinese boxes one within the other. There are the ever-shifting tides of experience and there is the changing focus of the Light which illumines them. Sometimes that focus is at one level, sometimes at another, and, wherever it is, that is the 'I', higher or lower as the case may be. To identify oneself with the Higher Ego means to focus the Light of Consciousness in the higher integrations of the psyche and to allow them to dominate the lower. At such moments the disciple is his Higher Self, or more accurately reflects it, since we are still dealing with a manifestation upon this lower plane of experience. At other times, when his consciousness is filled with feelings of I want, I wish and I dislike, it is the lower self which is holding the centre of the psyche's stage.

The verse concludes with the Guru's wish that he may find other disciples as firm in resolution as Nachiketas. Our mouths are always filled with complaints, or at least lamentations, about the difficulty of finding a true Guru but this is to look at things quite wrongly. There is in truth no difficulty in finding the Guru for "when the disciple is ready the Guru appears." The difficulty is in making ourselves adequate for discipleship. As always we project our inner difficulties on to the outer environment and blame the age we live in, the country we inhabit, or the social stratum in which we move for failures for which we and we alone are responsible. Now, as always, the Gurus are ready and waiting like the Buddha, of whom it is related that every morning he scanned the world with his Divine Eye to see if anywhere he could see one who had 'lit' his lamp, one who was ready to profit by the teaching.

No, it is not they who are difficult to find, but we who find it difficult to give ourselves to them, at least with that wholeness of self-giving which alone enables them to impart, or rather, *us to receive* the Teaching. Even if we have once given ourselves with some degree of what we know as wholeheartedness, we give ground under the fierce waves that inevitably assail us, "the evil that we would not, that we do" and thus have to echo the apostle's cry, "Who will deliver me from the body of this death?" To this cry there is only one answer; 'Not-I', an answer which underlies what theists know as the doctrine of grace and Far Eastern Buddhism as the doctrine of 'other power' as opposed to 'self power,'[1] two doctrines, however, which are as subtle as the edge of a razor—and as sharp to cut the hand. The words 'not-I' used above are also an explanation of our text's statement that when taught by 'another' the Wisdom is easy to be known.

Over the entrance to the Path is written in flaming letters "if thou hast any love of life, set not your foot on Me." .

(10) *I know that what is known as the Treasure-house is also impermanent; nor, in truth, is the Eternal to be gained by that which is temporal. Therefore by me has been laid the Nachiketas Fire and with transient things I have attained the Enduring.*

This verse has by some scholars been given to Nachiketas but that is not the traditional attribution and against it has been urged that we are not justified in making Nachiketas say that he had laid the Nachiketas

[1] *Tariki* and *Jiriki*. See any account of the *Amitābha*-invoking Schools of Japanese Buddhism.

Fire. This objection would not be insuperable if we wished to override it since neither the Fire is a literal one nor the real dialogue a half-hour affair. Nevertheless there seems no sound reason for departing from the traditional allocation of the verse to Yama.

The word *Shevadhi* rendered as Treasure-House has also other meanings for *sheva* means also a jewel, fish, serpent, male organ and a height or elevation. In fact it refers here to the great Treasure-House of the universe, the world of Brahma, the plane of *Mahat* or Cosmic Imagining. In it are garnered the treasures of Cosmic Experience, the Jewels of the point-like Higher Selves, the Fish of immortality, and the Serpents of Wisdom and unending cycles. The idea of the Serpent also suggests the enduring thread of the Higher Self on which, like beads, the separate personalities are strung, the *Sūtra-Ātman* or thread-Soul which again in some systems is a synonym for *Mahat*. The male organ, the pearl of great price to most of our modern psychologists, who, having once found it will go no further, is here a symbol of that creative ego-affirmation, the 'I' or Higher Self, which dwells in the bosom of its Father, the *Mahat*, which is, again, the Height or Elevation as opposed to the Depth here below. All these suggestions are contained in the word *Shevadhi* and are here drawn out so as to show what a wealth of meaning the archaic symbols contain as opposed to the modern paper currency with its ideal of one word, one meaning.

To understand this verse we must remember the teaching of the Nachiketas Fire and the 'immortality' of aeonian duration that is attained by it. He who has 'thrice' performed the fire sacrifice has passed beyond the realms of personal births and deaths and dwells as an Adept in the Great World or *Mahat*. As we have said before, he may or may not maintain a separate form on the lower levels, but, whether he does so or not, his true being remains rooted in what Greek initiates termed the Plain of Truth, the wide-stretching, all-embracing Cosmic Unity in which exist the Memories of all that has been, the 'plans' of all that is yet to be, the essential Life of all that now is. Hence is it called the Treasure-House.

Yet, says the Teacher, this Treasure-House with all its wealth which you are now able by means of the sacred Fire to attain is itself not permanent. True, it endures as long as the Cosmos of which it is the basis. Yet such aeonian endurance is not eternity, and it, with all that it contains, will be reabsorbed into the one Eternal at the coming of the Cosmic Night.

The true Eternal, the one fixed Star (*Dhruva* also means the pole star) round which the whole Cosmos turns, is not to be attained by means of anything which is itself non-eternal, that is to say, by anything which is part of the manifestation. The manifested cosmos in which are of course included all the higher worlds or planes of experience of which materialistic science knows nothing, is a many-dimensioned Whole of experience. In it may be drawn many patterns or out of it be constructed many dwellings. Some are constructed in one way and last but for a brief span. They are the dwellings of men. Others are constructed on a wider plan and endure for countless cycles. These are the dwellings of the Gods from which they watch with calm undisturbed eyes the birth and death of seas and mountain-chains and of the very worlds which bear them on their bosoms. Beyond these again, beyond the lake of Saturn and the 'Ageless' River, is the one great Palace, the Hall of Brahmā known as *Vibhu*, the Pervasive. In it are many wonders including the throne which is known as the Far-Shining (*Vichakshaṇā*) on which is seated Brahmā, "the Soul of every single living being."[1] This is the greatest dwelling of them all, the widest possible integration of cosmic experience, the farthest limit of manifested being, the many-mansioned House which includes all that is. Brahmā, the Life that ensouls this great dwelling is, as we have just quoted, the true Life of every living being and as such endures in wonderful pervading splendour during the countless ages of the Cosmic Day. Below him are the Gods and far below him men: during His mighty day, he sees the rise and set of universes. And yet this abiding Palace, this Treasure-House of which each of the countless worlds is but a brick, this world of Brahmā too, is not the one Eternal but only the greatest and most inclusive dwelling that can be constructed of the bricks of manifested being.

Beyond it is nothing, a Nothing which, like some invisible wall, obstructs the further passage of anything that is manifest, the Is or Is Not which is the subject of Nachiketas' third question, the mystic Nothingness which is the Source of all. To this eternal, nothing that is can be a means of attainment. Only by dropping everything can this Nothing be attained. Nor can any attain it, since, before attainment, he who would attain must cease to be.

"It is beyond you, because when you reach it you have lost your self. You will enter the light but you will never touch the Flame."

To the true mystic that Eternal Darkness which is the Light of Lights is as near to the ephemeral life of the lower world as it is to the exalted splendour of the world of Brahmā. Nevertheless, though there is in truth a door which leads from every house, even from the most ephemeral tenement, straight into It, yet it is a door which few can see and fewer open.

[1] For these symbols see Kaushitaki Upanishad I. 3-5.

79

Therefore, as the Teacher says, it is unwise to seek to leap at one bound across the ramparts. Rather, by skilful use of the ephemeral (remember that "Yoga is skill in action") we should seek to build up the altar for the Nachiketas Fire, and, with its aid, establish ourselves in that all-inclusive Dwelling which is referred to by Yama as the Enduring before attempting the final flight to the Alone. This is the so-much misunderstood path of *Krama-mukti* or liberation by stages. Shankara depreciated it in favour of the *Sadyo* or immediate liberation and most of those who follow the *Advaita Vedānta* have followed him—at least in theory. Whether they get satisfactory results in practice is a matter that can be left to them to judge, but we may remember the teaching of the Gita that "the difficulty of those whose minds are set on the Unmanifested is much greater. The (direct) way to the Unmanifest is indeed a hard one for those who are embodied."[1]

Much easier is it to climb step by step the Ladder of Being till the Great World of *Mahat* is reached whence the final flight to the Unmanifest Eternal can be made. This is the Path, the Path through the Great Being or *Vishwarūpa*, that Sri Krishna recommends, for it is this that is the meaning of the Universal Form which he showed to Arjuna in the eleventh chapter, and this that is the alternative mentioned by the latter in his question at the commencement of the twelfth.

This is why Yama says *therefore* the Nachiketas Fire has been made use of by him. Faced by the difficulty that on the direct Path to the Unmanifested, as Plotinus said, *all* forms, whether of sense or whether

---

[1] Gita 12. 5; Cf. also "The secret of the magic of life consists in using action in order to achieve inaction. One must not wish to leave out the steps between and penetrate directly." *Secret of the Golden Flower.*

of thought, have to be abandoned, and knowing how almost impossible that is for us who, whether we wish or no, are rooted in the sense life, he recommends the gradual Path on which the transient experiences of life are transmuted by the Sacred Fire and thus made use of as the means of ascent.

For, as the Gita again teaches us, the One Eternal *is* present even in the most trivial experiences of life: "The all-pervading *Brahman* stands ever in the Cosmic sacrifice" which is life.[1] By "skill in action," then, by making an offering of all experience in the Inner Fire of sacrifice, we can make the gradual ascent and "by means which are transient, attain the Enduring," or, as the Tantras put it, "by those things by which men fall, by those very things shall they rise."

Those who wish to make further study of this Path are referred to the Gita of which it is in a very special sense the subject matter.[2] Our present Upanishad is more directly concerned with what the alchemists termed the "Philosophic Work," the transmutation of the mental view itself without which the 'Metallic Work' or physical transmutation cannot be accomplished. Here, then, we shall only say briefly that on this Path every act, every thought and every feeling is directed towards the one loved Figure, who, whether He be the personal Teacher, a symbolic form of the inner Guru or the figure of the Divine *avatāra*, is in reality a symbol of the Universal Self. In this way even the pettiest details of life become elements in a sacrifice. The self-reference in which lies their binding power is destroyed in the Fire of Love. "For love he acts, for love he speaks and thinks, and so by love he rises swiftly to the Goal. Where there is love no sacri-

[1] *Gita* 3.15.
[2] See my *Yoga of the Bhagawat Gita.*

fice can be too great to be performed with joy......Here is the power lying in all men's hearts by which to scale the peaks of the Eternal."[1]

Nevertheless we must also remember that the Universal Soul, the Great Being of the Brahma-World, is not itself the Eternal but only the farthest limit of manifestation. Nachiketas seeks the ultimate knowledge of That which is beyond all manifestations and therefore Yama continues:

(11) *Thou, O Nachiketas, art wise; for having seen the fulfilment of all desire, the Foundation of the world, the infinity of creative will, the fearless other Shore, the Great One, mantra-bodied* (stomam), *the Wide-extended, that in which all is established, thou hast with firmness put* (*this great attainment*) *from thee.*[2]

The danger in the Path of Gradual Liberation (and there are inevitably dangers on *every* path) one, that perhaps underlies Shankara's depreciation of it, is that aspirants are apt to mistake the attainment of some relatively lofty stage for the final Goal and to rest content with that. In the Gita, too, Sri Krishna tells his pupil that the true Yogi, having known the states that

---

[1] *Yoga of the Bhagawat Gita*, p. 115.

[2] Dr. Coomaraswami has some particularly interesting notes on this verse which, however, arrived too late to be noticed in the text. His interpretation depends on giving a different meaning, that of 'emanation', to the word *atyasrākshiḥ* here rendered, following the general usage, as 'abandoned' or 'put away.' This involves a similar alteration, though not so serious a one, in verse 3 where the same word is used. Partly because the said notes arrived too late and partly because I do not regard the case for alteration as altogether proved, I have left my own version unchanged but if established it is perhaps worthy of note that it would offer a very interesting parallel to the alchemical 'Powder of Projection', i. e., of emanation as suggested.

result from sacrifice, alms and good deeds, passes them all by and soars beyond them to the "Supreme and Primeval Abode."[1]

Moreover, the real Power by which the ascent is to be made is the one secret Power, the power of the One Eternal that is hidden in the heart. That Power can only effectively be drawn on by one whose aspiration is towards the Eternal, one who can echo the words of the Orphic initiate "pure I go to the pure." Lesser aspirations are all very well in their way but at best they give a slow and halting progress, the Way of the Ant, as it was known in ancient India. The real soaring flight, the Way of the Eagle, can only be achieved by drawing on the hidden Power of the Eternal, the power "which shall make him appear as nothing in the eyes of men", the power of the mystic Nothingness, the hidden Void.

A sense of false modesty which is really only a lurking and negative egoism may urge the disciple to take some lower attainment as his immediate goal saying that when he reaches it he will then think of going farther. But this, like all that has its roots in the ego, is a snare. Not only is the Eternal the only true Goal, in a very real sense it is also the Path to that Goal and the strength by which the Path is trod. No flight that is not winged by that secret strength can do more than skim feebly over the surface of the earth. He who would soar to Heaven must use Heaven's wings.[2]

It is for this reason that the teacher praises Nachiketas for refusing to be satisfied with any lesser attainment, however lofty, even with the sublime attainment of the Universal Being, for this it is to which the

---

[1] *Gita* 8. 28.

[2] This is a topic we shall have to return to later in this chapter.

epithets in this verse apply.

It is the Fulfilment of all desire because it is the All. The movements of desire arise from the sense of separateness. Where, as in this Brahma World, all is one harmonious whole, desire can have no place, for all that is unintelligently sought outside itself is here attained. In this divine state the circumference of one is the Circumference of All. It is the Foundation, not only of this, but of all worlds, for it is the Whole out of which by abstraction they are formed, the Matrix in which even now they have their being.

It is the Infinity of Creative Will because it is the ultimate dynamism of the universe, at least as far as manifested being is concerned. The whole Power of the Eternal, polarised as it is into the Sun and Moon, is focussed in this Divine Son who partakes of both. It is a living Norm which regulates all movements in the lower worlds. Its enduring archetypal harmony becomes, when reflected in the worlds of time and change, the living Will which directs all movements in them. In it is centred the Creative Power which wields the stars and planets in the sky and also the atoms and electrons of which those stars are made.

> "It maketh and unmaketh, mending all;
> What it hath wrought is better than had been;
> Slow grows the splendid pattern that it plans;
> Its wistful hands between."[1]

It is the Fearless Other Shore, because, though within the manifested universe, it is beyond the sorrowful worlds of change, those levels of being on which birth and death take place, on which the planets whirl in chains around their central suns. It is beyond the flowing stream of time as known to us; fearless because

[1] *Light of Asia.*

within its bosom separation, the parent of all fear, is absent. In it each mingles with each and in each is found the All. As has been said elsewhere: "Where there is duality there is fear of another but where all is the Self what should there be to fear?"

The Great one is a reference to the term by which it is commonly known in the philosophical systems (especially in the Sānkhya) namely *Mahat*. With this term goes *Urugāya*, the Wide-Extended, which can also be rendered as the Wide-Striding, a reference to the famous three Strides of Vishnu, for Vishnu, as the Pervader, the one manifested Self of all, strides through the Three Worlds of change and sorrow and is established in the Fourth, that "Supreme Standing Place which is ever beheld by the Sages extended like the Eye of Heaven."[1]

Less obvious perhaps is the meaning of the epithet *Stomam* which we have rendered Mantra-bodied. The word *stoma* literally means a vedik 'hymn,' a mantra or collection of mantras. Most readers will be familiar with the term *Shabda Brahman*, the Sound-Brahman, a term which is also applied to the Vedas, or collections of mantras. This *Shabda Brahman* is essentially the same as the *Mahat*, the Great one. It is the Great Word, the creative Logos, the Pythagorean Harmony of the Spheres. In the Kabala it is the famous Jod-He-Vau-He, the sacred four-lettered Name of God, the fundamental power in all beneficent magic. Those fortunate ones whose keen vision has penetrated to this Divine World know well the Mystic and tremendous Sound that pulses through eternity as Changeless Being

---

[1] Using another scale of reference this Fourth is of course the Unmanifest beyond even the *Mahat*. These ancient symbols can be applied on more than one scale, a fact which has been a source of great confusion to scholars.

85

manifests in change. Some also will remember the fiery letters that flash over the Deep, letters in which the living Powers of mantra symbolically body themselves forth to the eye of the Seer.[1]

That great Sound, the *Mahā Mantra*, is the beating of the Mighty Cosmic Heart and its awe-inspiring reverberations are around us now and forever. So deaf are our ears, however, that, as Pythagoras said, we are unable to hear it. "Having ears we hear not." Those who can hear it know that it is the Root of all the sounds we hear, the fundamental Rhythm into which blend in a wonderful harmony every single one of the many differing rhythms we know in our life down here. The voice of the winds in forests, the deep and sliding murmur of great rivers, the thunder of the waves on rocky coasts, the living beating of our hearts, yes, and the ticking of clocks and the so-called dead pulse of a liner's engines; all these are echoes of that one great Sound out of which they grow, forming the elements of one harmonious Pattern. All that we know as sounds or movements are in fact the manifestations of that timeless Rhythm in time. What is termed *mantra-yoga* is a use of sounds, as in other yogas visualised forms or mental concepts are used, to form a ladder by which the ascent may be made from the gross to the subtle and from the subtle to the deep Divine.

Lastly, it is the *Pratishṭhā*, the Establishment, for it is that in which all manifestation, whether of 'Matter' or of 'Form' is rooted, out of which it emerges and in which, however seeming separate, even now it has its real being.

Why then if this Brahma-world, the *Hiranyagarbha* or Golden Womb, as Shankara terms it, is all this that

---

[1] It was no 'mere' poetic license, no milk and water metaphor that made the Vedik seers talk of *seeing* the mantras.

we have said, should Yama praise Nachiketas for putting it from him ? One reason we have already given; another may now be added. As may be seen from a perusal of the above epithets, the Brahma-world is the Land of Heart's Desire, for all the terms used above can be applied also to the natural desires of man. *Stoma* thus means praise, *Urugāya* wide and kingly dominion (cf., the offer in 1. 23) and *pratishṭhā*, 'establishment' in the worldly sense. All these desires of the heart have their fulfilment in the Brahma-world and any aspiration towards the latter that is not winged with utter renunciation of all such is fettered by chains of desire, however golden. The Golden Womb is indeed the Fulfilment of Desire (*Kāmasyāptim*) but he who seeks it because of that will never find the trackless Swan's Path that leads Beyond.

(12) *Having known by means of the union with the Inner Self* (adhyātma yoga), *that Shining Power, very difficult to see, present in the Darkness, dwelling in the Cavern of the Heart, abiding in the Abyss, Primaeval, the wise one abandons joy and sorrow.*

(13) *Having heard and thoroughly grasped this, (and) having picked out and obtained the subtle Monad, the Bearer of the (manifest) qualities,*[1] *the mortal rejoices having attained the House of Bliss.*[2] *For Nachiketas, I think, the Dwelling is open.*[3]

---

[1] *Dharmyam* here signifies the bearer of the *dharmas* or qualities, i.e., the one Reality which appears as variously qualified. Cf. 4. 14.

[2] Literally "That which is to be rejoiced in."

[3] Thus, both Shankara and Madhva: some modern translators prefer to render the last sentence as "I consider Nachiketas an open (or opened) dwelling" which, if accepted, would refer to the house of the Body which has been 'opened' by the liberated. Compare the words of the Buddha:—"Never again shalt thou, O builder of

Other than the Path leading to the Brahma-
world, though passing through that same world, is the
Path that leads to the Eternal. Its gateway lies, as the
Buddha also taught, "within this fathom-long human
form." Ordinary life is the *adhibhautika yoga*, the union
with the objects of sense which lie around us in the outer
world. Uniting with those objects, we share their
perishable nature. Embarking with our Gold in leaky
ships, we sink with them and tread the path of darkness.
Opposed to this is the *Adhyātmayoga*, the union with what
is of the nature of the self, the shining Light of the consciousness within. When we turn away from the brightly
lit sense world and look within ourselves we at first
find nothing but darkness—Russell, I believe, has somewhere contrasted the rich world outside with the sterile
darkness within. But what is night to the ordinary man
is day to the seer and within that darkness is a shining
and divine Power, the Light of all the worlds, the one
Light of all seeing whatsoever. Used as we are to
attending only to what is seen, it is at first difficult to
realise the presence of that Seer, He who having entered
into the darkness of outwardness known symbolically
as Matter dwells in the Abyss, the Cavern that is in the
heart of man.

Before going further, let us pause a moment over
this famous Cavern. The usual modern comment—
how often have we not heard it—is that the ancient
peoples, ignorant of the functions of the brain, believed
the seat of consciousness to be the heart. It is not so;
the facts are quite the other way round. It was not the
ancient seers but the moderns who display ignorance, for

houses, make a house again for me: broken are all thy beams, thy
ridge pole shattered." But it seems hardly correct to consider
Nachiketas at this stage as one who has "finished the course"
and it would only be for such a one that the interpretation
would hold.

the latter imagine that they know all about the heart when they have called it a blood-pump and can talk learnedly about ventricles, valves and what not.

If we are to talk of a seat of consciousness at all, or rather of the psyche which includes far more than what we know as consciousness, it is perfectly correct to place that seat in the heart. The heart is the correlative on the physical scale of being of the fundamental psychic centre and may thus be termed its vehicle or seat. Moreover, there *are* caverns in it, even physical caverns, as every six penny text-book writer knows, and these caverns are in truth Caverns of the Winds as is testified to by the very name of 'ventricle.' From these Caverns issue the four Winds of Heaven, both those which whisper gently in pine-forests and those which are now raging hurricane-like in Europe. Also in the heart, whether anatomists have found it or not, is the deep Well, from which comes bubbling up the spring of Life, the Well which is also the Well of Truth, the Deep Abyss hidden in which, as our verse tells us, abides the Primaeval Spirit of Light. No; it was most assuredly not 'ignorance' that led the Seers to speak as they did of the Heart. The brain and its consciousness is a mere upstart usurper like the Gnostic Ildabaoth who boastfully exclaimed, "I am Father and God and beyond me is no other," till his mother, the Wisdom, rebuked him saying, "Lie not, Ildabaoth, for above thee is the All Father, the first Man and Man the Son of Man." A saying which is reported to have "astonished all the Powers" just as it astonishes the 'powers' of our present world.[1]

[1] *Fragments of a Faith Forgotten* by G. R. S. Mead, p. 189. Compare also: "The lower heart moves like a strong, powerful commander who despises the Heavenly Ruler because of his weakness and has seized for himself the leadership of the affairs of state." *The Secret of the Golden Flower* transl. by Wilhelm.

The Yoga of the Kaṭhopaniṣad

The Indian Gurus, from the earliest Vedik seers who proclaimed that it was by searching in the heart that they had discovered "the existents' kinship in the Non-existent" to those of today, have rightly taught that he who would tread the Path must seek within the heart for its Door. In the very centre of the four Caverns is to be found the sacred Well of whose water he who drinks "shall never thirst again." From those deep waters, so dark at first, issues a Light which we had not noticed, the blue light that illuminates the Caverns. From time to time a Spirit troubles them as it troubled long ago the Healing Pool of Siloam, a luminous spray is seen on the surface and from depths below arises a hand "clothed in white samite, mystic, wonderful," holding amidst the spray the Magic Emblem which will serve as talisman and key. It is at such moments, and if not watched for they will pass before we are ready to take advantage of them, that we must spring boldly, and, grasping the magic talisman, dive deep in one clean plunge. Not at the first attempt does any reach the Depths. He who has gained them has abandoned joy and sorrow.

The Upanishad goes on to say that he who has heard this from a competent Teacher, has heard it, as the old magical teaching puts it, "with the understanding of the heart," and can seize the subtle central Point (*aṇu*), the *Dharmya* or Bearer of the qualities and images that we call objects, whose arm it was that held the mystic symbol, such a one will rejoice in the unbroken bliss of the Eternal, the bliss that fills the Home within the Waters. For the true disciple that Home stands ever open.

Perhaps we shall be told that we have darkened the text. Those who think that must seek for light elsewhere. We can only repeat; a hand emerges from the Waters of Life and in it is a symbol. Grasp that symbol and seek resolutely for him who holds it. The

90

Arm is a long one but he who finds its Body has found the Goal. These instructions are perfectly plain for those for whom they are intended and no attempt will be made to change them into the thin paper currency of the conscious mind, a currency the spurious clarity of which can be more utterly misleading than the darkest oracles of ancient speech.

Not for paper money will the Ferry-man of the Dead carry over the Soul in his boat, nor will saccharine tablets serve as a substitute for the honeycake with which Cerberus, the Watcher by the Door must be appeased.[1]

(14) *Other than* Dharma, *other than* Adharma; *other than both Cause and Effect; other also than Past and Future; That which thou seest, tell me that.*

The question in this verse is traditionally ascribed to Nachiketas though there are no signs in the verse itself warranting the attribution except the bare fact that it is a question. Accordingly some modern translators put it into the mouth of Yama and regard it as a rhetorical question. Perhaps it would be even

---

[1] This Ferry-man, the Charon of Greek teaching is similar to the Non-human being, the *amānava Purusha*, who in the *Chhāndogya Upanishad* is described as leading the Souls along the Pathway of the Gods. In the Greek myth he had to be given a coin which was accordingly placed by friends in the mouth of the dead. For the same reason gold is placed in the mouth of the dead in India. A similar figure was Hermes Psychopompos, Hermes the guide of the Souls, who held in his hands "a beautiful golden Rod" with which he "spell-binds the eyes of the dead and wakes them again too from sleep, those namely who become mindful" (See the Naasene Teachings). Cerberus, the three-headed dog who guards the Halls of Death, corresponds to the two four-eyed Hounds of Yama, who sit as guardians on the path. We may remember also the Jackal headed Anubis who was the guide of Souls in Egypt and who was combined with Hermes in the form of Hermanubis.

truer to regard it as one of those questions that are asked of the disciple by the Guru and which serve the former as a subject on which to concentrate his mind until the answer is found. An example may be found in the Tibetan *Yoga of the Great Symbol.*[1] Similar, though with a characteristic difference, is the *Koan* of Zen Buddhism in Japan. Such questions are an extremely useful technique, at least for a certain type of disciple. The problem is set, and, day after day the disciple revolves it in his mind until his thought becomes saturated with it and it is present even in his dreams. Then, when the mind falls back exhausted and baffled (and the question set is deliberately of a baffling sort, even, may be, one to which no answer in intellectual terms can be given) the answer flashes from the deeper levels of the psyche and, then, not only is the particular problem solved, but, what is more important, the disciple has learnt how to open the Door that leads to Knowledge.

In the present case the question is one which refers to the nature of the absolutely unqualified, the Transcendent. In this universe everything is in motion: indeed the word *Jagat* or world means the moving thing. Of these motions, whether on the physical, emotional, or mental levels of experience, we can distinguish two sorts, one of which is in harmony with the Norm or Cosmic Harmony, the *Ṛita*, while the second is distorted and inharmonious. These two are known respectively as *Dharma* and *Adharma*. The former

---

[1] "What is the real nature of the 'Non Moving' (or mind when it is motionless)?

How it remaineth motionless?

Whether the 'Moving' is other than the Non-moving?

How the 'Moving' becometh the non-moving?"

Translated by Dr. Evans Wentz and Lama Dawa Samdup in '*Tibetan Yoga and Secret Doctrines.*'

comprises all such actions or movements in general as reflect the *Ṛita*, the eternal norm "laid up in the heavens" of the *Mahat*. Such movements are termed *Dharma*, and, being harmonious, they set up no strain anywhere.

The universe, however, is not a machine, not something which rolls inexorably along predestined grooves with perfect predictability. The light of Consciousness is free with the essential freedom of the *Atman*, and, though that freedom is more and more limited the deeper we descend into matter, it can never be annulled. On no level whatsoever are movements compelled to be in harmony with the Cosmic Pattern and thus we need feel no surprise at the modern scientific 'discovery' that even the movements of electrons are not strictly determined.

Free as the Soul is, however, to take its own line, it can never escape the normative pull of the Harmony, any self-willed divergence from the lines of which sets up a strain in the psychic continuum or Ambient, a strain that is just as real as that produced by pulling on one side of a rubber sheet. That strain produces its effect upon the acting centre, the 'self,' human or non-human, and that effect serves to compensate unerringly for the one-sidedness, the disharmony of the action. Such a self-willed unharmonious action is known as *adharma*: the compensating effect due to the strain set up is termed *karma*, the fruit of actions, 'the law' by which "the slayer's knife did stab himself," by which, in fact, all actions "like chickens, return home to roost."

It goes without saying that all movements in this universe fall into one of these two classes. Where, however, there is a duality, a pair of polar opposites, there is certainly a unity which underlies the two poles. What is that unity ?

Again, we have another pair of poles, those of cause and effect. We are accustomed to discriminate all phenomena as either causes or effects though it is obvious that what is cause from one point of view is effect from another. Moreover, as the disciple advances on this Path, he comes to see that there is no true causation at all but only correlation on this physical plane. "The things that act upon each other are branchings from a far-off beginning and so stand distinct; but they derive initially from the one source: all interaction is like that of brothers, resemblant as drawing life from the same parents."[1] The same teaching is set forth by the great Agrippa: "There is therefore no other cause of the necessity of effects than the connection of all things with the First Cause and their correspondency with those Divine Patterns and Eternal Ideas whence everything hath its determinate and particular place in the exemplary world."[2] All the movements that we see happen around us are in reality but effects whose causes are to be sought in those higher worlds from which the lower hang, the levels that are known in Indian thought as Causal (*Kāraṇa*). Nevertheless, we still have our polarity, though now a vertical instead of a horizontal one. What is that which is beyond both cause and effect ?

Once more we can look at the movements in relation to what we call time. Here we find the knife-edge of the present, in which alone movements *are*, dividing the past in which similar movements *have been* from a future in which they *will be*. Yet the past still exists in some sense for its movements still affect us, and, as Plato said, existence means power to act. In similar, though perhaps less obvious ways, the future too affects us now and it is well known to all but those who will not see that "coming events cast their shadows before."

[1] Plotinus 3. 3. 7.
[2] Cornelius Agrippa *Three Books on Occult Philosophy*.

Chapter II

What then is that mysterious existence which is beyond
the categories of past and future, that exists in an eternal
present ?

Those are the questions that the pupil is set to
solve, the solution of which will open for him the Door.
The answer, which comprises the rest of the Upanishad,
may be regarded as declared by Yama when Nachiketas
remained silent or as being the answer which sprang
up in the latter's heart as a result of his brooding concentration on the questions. The two alternatives are
in reality the same, since Yama, as we have seen, is the
Higher self of the disciple and it is from that Higher
Self that the answer comes, whether through the lips
of an embodied Teacher or through those other lips
that speak soundlessly in the disciple's heart. As the
Upanishad itself will tell us later: "He who sees difference here will go from death to death."

(15) *That word which all the Vedas declare, which all
inward-turnings* (tapānsi) *sound forth, desiring which men lead
the Mystic Life* (Brahmacharyam): *that Word I tell thee
briefly: It is Om.*

The term we have translated as Word is *Padam*
which is pregnant with many other meanings such as
path, goal, abode, and also, significantly enough, a
ray of light. All of these meanings have to be kept
in mind. We have chosen to render it as Word because
it is in the form of a mystic word that the *padam* is set
forth and because it corresponds to what the Graeco-
Egyptian mystics referred to as the Logos, the formative divine Utterance which gives pattern to the cosmos.
Its identification by scholastic writers with the principle
of 'Reason' arose because the faculty known to us by
that name is essentially the ordering and pattern-making
faculty in our world. Nevertheless to equate the two

is to take the part, and a very small part at that, for the whole.

This Word, then, or Logos, is the one central Principle round which revolves all the rich symbolism of the Vedas as unerringly as the starry heavens revolve round the Pole-star, also, incidentally, called a *padam*. By Vedas we must here understand not only the books so known in India, but the entire body of sacred teachings all over the world. The Veda, from the root *vida*, means the Knowledge and all such knowledge is concerned with the knowing of one central Principle "which having known there is nothing more here that needs to be known."[1]

This same Logos is also sounded forth by all acts of what is known as *tapasya*, often translated as austerity, but really meaning the brooding warmth, the secret inner Fire, that is generated by turning the consciousness inward towards its source, what is nowadays termed introversion and which in one form or another, is the source of all magical power. By such *tapasya*, such inner Fire, we read elsewhere, the universe itself burst forth from the brooding *Brāhmik* being. All such inward-turning sounds forth the Word with all its magical creative power.

The word *Brahmacharyam* again, which has nowadays come to mean simply sexual restraint, had originally a far wider import. It was the name for the life lived by the pupil at the feet of his Guru, and, since the word *Brahma* means both the great and also the mystical or sacred, we have given it its fundamental meaning of the inner or mystic life. All other meanings are, once more, a taking of the part for the whole. It is easy to see how they arose, for the very essence of that inner path lies in self-restraint, and, among the various

---

[1] *Gita* 7. 2.

types of such, sexual restraint is the one which looms largest in the mind of the ordinary man. To restrain the sex impulses is for him restraint *par excellence* (in the same way as 'immorality' usually means just sexual irregularity) and the other equally important restraints, restraint of temper, for instance, are apt to be more or less completely ignored.

In any case, the knowledge of the Sacred Word is the real goal round which centres the whole of the Inner Life.

That word is Om.

(16) *This Word is indeed the Brahman. This Word is indeed the Supreme. Whatever he desires is his who knows this Word.*

(17) *This is the best means (of attainment); This is the highest Support.[1] Having known this Support one becomes great in the Brahma-World.*

In these two verses the Teacher goes on to extol the greatness of the Unique Word. The 'word' of the first verse is not, as before, *padam*, but *aksharam* which signifies, in addition to word or syllable, the Imperishable. Similarly in the second verse *ālambanam* means a support, that from which anything hangs, and also, by a special application of this idea, a 'support' for meditation, a springboard, as it were, from which to plunge into the Waters that are beyond the mind. Such 'support' may be of many kinds, a visual form, a sound

[1] The same word *ālambanam* signifies both a support and also a means of attainment: hence the word has been translated differently in the two lines. Note also the play of words in the last line of verse 17 where the word *Mahīyate*, literally is honoured, embodies a reference to the *Mahat* with which the soul becomes identified.

or an idea.   Here the *Om* is stated to be the best of all such.

The exposition of the *Praṇava* (*Om*) is contained in the *Māṇḍūkya Upanishad*.   It is a subject in itself and we cannot go into it in any detail here.   Something, however, must be said about the reasons for its special excellence as a 'support' for meditation.

In the first place it affords a convenient combination of all three of the types of mental support previously mentioned.   It is at once a visual form, ॐ, a sound, and an idea or rather combination of ideas.   Its mono-syllabic unity divides into three elements A, U, M, which, together with what is sometimes called the *Ardha-mātrā* or echoing half-beat, symbolise the three worlds and the unmanifest Fourth.   More elaborate analyses, including a seven-fold one, are also known but the above is the most usual and convenient.

Again, it epitomises the entire gamut of vocal sounds for it commences with the A sound produced at the back of the throat and finishes with closed lips for the M.

Still again, if pronounced in a particular manner, it is an approximation to the Great Sound to which we have already referred and of which it is the symbol.

For all these reasons it is the great mantra of the Vedik tradition and as such is prefixed to all other man-tras.[1]   In fact we may say that the other mantras are only a drawing out and a rendering more comprehensible of the meanings contained in the *Om*.   As such, when the pupil has advanced a certain distance, he is allowed to drop them and retain only the *Om* which is thus the essence of all the Vedas.

Not only is it a symbol of the dual *Brahman*, the

---

[1] Vedik mantras, that is; the tantric tradition while not ignoring the *Om*, makes use of other sounds as well as and sometimes instead of it.

manifested *Brahman* which is this universe and the unmanifested *Brahman* beyond: it is also an expression or manifestation of it, for all true and living symbols are manifestations of that which they symbolise. This is what differentiates them, in fact, from the artificialities of mere allegory. Hence, says the Teacher, it can itself be spoken of as the *Brahman* and is not only the best support for meditation but is also itself That which is the Support of all.

It is in itself, at once the Supreme, the one Eternal, the Great Sound of the Brahma-world, and also the three lower worlds of birth and death. With *Om* the universe was breathed forth, with *Om* it is maintained in being now and with *Om* it will be again withdrawn at the end of the Cosmic Day.

With *Om* the Heavenly Sphere with all its stars and planets revolves around the earth,[1] with *Om* rise and fall the waves of that Leaden Sea we call the solid land, with *Om* the rivers flow towards the ocean and with *Om* that ocean beats for ever on the land. With *Om*, too, the hosts of men rush forth to battle, with *Om* they clash together and again with *Om* they leave their outer shells to tread an unseen path.

He who with knowledge can utter the *Om* can certainly, as the verse says, gain whatever he desires, for in it is the whole power of the creative Logos.

We must hasten to add, however, that by correct utterance is not meant any mere pronunciation that can be learnt by studying the throat and lip movements of another man. Not by mere instruction as a later verse tells us is the utterance to be learnt nor will any known science of phonetics avail to write it down.

---

[1] Quite, quite ! we have not forgotten Copernicus, but all motion is relative. Modern scientists will tell us that the Copernican or heliocentric description is *simpler* rather than truer. Simpler for certain purposes no doubt: not so for others.

The word must be uttered not with lips alone but with the whole fourfold being of the psyche if it is to manifest the creative Power which we have described above. It is in the heart that we must utter it or rather must unite with its eternal utterance, for no man can pronounce it but only 'God' himself. In the very centre it wells up, a throbbing fountain of Sound which rolls echoing around the deep Caverns, impressing itself on their walls in ten thousand hieroglyphic forms which contain for him who can read them all knowledge, human and divine. We walk this earth in dark and pitiable ignorance and yet we bear within our breasts the secret rock-cut library in which is stored the ageless Secret Knowledge. That which our scientists will or will not, millennia hence, 'discover' is written now upon those cavern walls though few indeed are they who can read even the elements of the writing; those who master it in its entirety live no more as men among us.

(18) *This Knower is not born nor does he die. Nor from anywhere has he become anything. Unborn Enduring, Everlasting and Primordial, he is not killed in the killing of the body.*

(19) *If the slayer thinks to slay or the slain thinks he is slain, neither of them know the truth. This (Knower) neither slays nor is slain.*

The term *Vipaschit*, which, following the general usage and dictionary meaning, we have translated as the Knower, the Wise One, the Soul, comes from the root *Vip*, meaning to vibrate. We can thus see why it is that out of dozens of possible terms, this particular one should have been used here to denote the Soul. The *Vipaschit* means he whose consciousness vibrates in harmony with the *Om* of which it is the knower. Only thus can we see the connection between these verses and the previous ones. We have been told that all desires are his who knows the *Om* and that he unites his being with the deathless *Brāhmik* being of the *Mahat*. We have also said that none can utter the *Om* but can only unite his being with its perpetual utterance. The consciousness (*chit*) of him who does so is thus assimilated to the Cosmic Rhythm and so may be said to vibrate along with it and to become a moment of the great *Brāhmik* Being, the Universal Soul, the mighty rhythm of which now manifests through his heart.

United with that Being, he partakes knowingly in its immortality. He knows that winter no less than summer, night no less than day, 'death' no less than 'life' are but the phases of that rhythm, the thoughts and crests of its unceasing waves. He becomes aware that however the cyclic seasons come and go there is no death for him. He is as much present in the dark withdrawn life of winter as in the exuberant out-pouring of the summer. Knowing the *Om*, he accepts both of these as equal aspects of his being. Bodies arise and decay but he neither rises with them nor decays with their decay. Not he in them but they in him. From nowhere has he come, for he stands forever in his own enduring being, apart from all comings and goings. Nor is there anywhere where he can go, since there is nowhere that is outside himself. Nor is there anything he can become: he is the All. His light illumines forms and the ignorant say he has become those forms. But he has no more become them than the sunlight has become the objects that it shines upon.

Forms come and go in his light but they are no more him than the passing gestures we make with our hands, the words which issue from our lips, are 'us.' They take place in our being and serve us for expression but we never feel that we have ceased to be because the word which we utter comes to an end. So with the *vipaschit*. His bodies are the words he utters, linked together in long strings of which no single one comprehends the meaning of the whole series. Yet when the series is complete the meaning of the whole stands forth plain for all to see. Each word stands by itself as an independent entity and yet the meaning of each is bound up with those that have gone before and with those that will succeed it in the sentence.

He is the Eternal, the enduring Speaker, coeval with the Universe of which he is the Logos. Night follows day and day follows night in endless succession but he neither comes nor goes with them. All is within his being, all moves according to the Rhythm which is himself. How indeed should he be slain by the destruction of a body? He slays not neither is he ever slain.   .

(20) *Smaller than the small, greater than the great is the* Ātman *that dwells in the secret heart* (guhāyām) *of beings. He who is free from desire, by tranquillity of the senses beholds that Greatness of the* Ātman *(and becomes) freed from sorrow.*[1]

He who has known the *Om*, knows indeed that it is within all things. The vibrations of the tiniest atoms or electrons as much as the whirlings of the vastest Cosmic nebulae are expressions of the one great Rhythm. It is the power which draws them forth, supports them in their movements and into which again they are dis-

---

[1] Some texts—at any rate some translators—read *dhātuḥ pra-sādāt* instead of *dhātu prasādāt* thus making it into "by the grace of the Creator (*dhātri*)." I have followed Shankara in reading by "the tranquillity of the senses," a reading which is far more to the point and far more in harmony with the tenor, not only of this, but of all the other early Upanishads.

solved. In truth, it is not within them any more than the sun actually rises and sets. They are in It not It in them but such is the force of habit that we can but talk of it as being within them. Indeed it is their very core, the heart of their being. It is the Light itself, they are its waves. Neither microscope nor telescope can compass its being. Cleave the minutest atom, it is there: mount to the outer space beyond all stars; still we are within its all-enfolding arms. It is the Wondrous Being, the Dragon of Life and Wisdom. It soars majestic in the heavens and the starry worlds play like fire-flies beneath the shadow of its outspread wings, and yet, at the same time, it dwells in the subtle central Well that is in the midst of the Caverns of the heart, the well that is subtler than "the hundredth part of a hair." He is the *Atman*, the 'Breath,' that blows the bubbles of the worlds.[1]

The text goes on to tell us how we may behold that Wondrous Greatness. First and foremost we must abandon desire, since it is the force of desire that is for ever taking us outside ourselves, away from the mystic Centre of our being in which the *Atman* dwells. Again and again desire lures us forth to seek outside ourselves what is only to be gained within. Again and again we sink back, satiate or frustrated: "vanity of vanities all is vanity." But it is only for a moment and the next wave that comes along once more carries us with it into the waters of outwardness, the bitter sea of sorrow.

He who would see the Greatness of the *Atman* must first learn to stand unmoved by those surging waves, and, to do this, he must first learn how it is that they succeed in carrying him away. The senses are the limbs by which those waves take hold of us, or, to

---

[1] The root meaning of *Atman*, as of the Greek *pneuma*, is breath.

change the symbolism, they are the sails by which the
wind seizes hold of the boat of the Soul. "Such of the
roving senses as the mind yields to, carry off its wisdom
as the wind a ship upon the waters."[1]

Hence the first step is to lower those sails so that
the soul's boat can remain poised on the swelling waves,
serenely riding out the blowing gales. In other words
the consciousness must cease to identify itself with the
senses. It must detach itself from them so that they remain calm and tranquil, the flame of light burning
straight and clear "like a lamp in a windless place."
Only when this has been accomplished will the mind
cease to be carried away by desire and be able, as
Patanjali says, "to stand in its own nature" and to perceive that what it had thought to be the light of day
outside itself was but a moonlight reflected from the
true Sunlight of the *Ātman* within. Beholding the greatness of that Light within itself, it ceases utterly to desire
anything that is without. No more will it leap forth in
frenzied pursuit of what it has not got: no more will
it experience the anger of frustration, the weary satiety
of illusive possession. Instead it beholds the serene
and all-encompassing Light. Within it is all, all that
it vainly sought without. Harbour is reached, the sails
are dropped. Desire has disappeared, and, with desire, all sorrow.

(21) *Seated he travels far; lying he goes in all directions.
Who but me is able to know that Shining One who rejoices and
rejoices not ?*

(22) *Bodiless within the bodies, stable amidst the unstable,
having known the great and all-pervading* Ātman, *the wise
one sorrows no more.*

---

[1] *Gītā* 2. 67.

Chapter II

Ordinary speech, based as it is on the notions of separateness, is unable to describe the wonderful nature of the *Atman* except by the use of symbol and paradox, for symbol directly involves the intuitive *buddhi* beyond the mind and paradox, by insisting on the simultaneous presence of what to the reason are contraries, does the same. The marvellous living omnipresence of the *Atman* has to be experienced to be grasped. No mere metaphor, based on our ordinary experience, is adequate. If we say that it resembles *ākāsha* or space we shall get a wrong idea, since, *to our thought*, the omnipresence of space is a dead or static one and there is nothing static about the *Atman*. Yet when we say there is nothing static we are again wrong for it is essentially that which stands for ever. With us when a thing stands it is not moving and *vice versa*, but the *Atman* is beyond these opposites. It stands forever, unmoved amid the moving, and yet it moves with a speed infinitely beyond that of light. The latter takes eight minutes to reach us from the sun and many many years to travel from the distant stars. Not so the *Atman* which girdles the Universe in one instantaneous flash, and all without moving from its original position. We are reminded of the story of the Buddha, pursued by the dacoit Angulimāla. However hotly the latter pursued, he could by no means come nearer. Exhausted, he called out to the Buddha to stand still; whereupon the Buddha replied, "I am standing: do thou also stand."

Therefore the Teacher, making use of paradox tells us that though seated firmly in one place, the *Atman* yet travels far, though lying in perfect repose it moves everywhere, and he asks "who other than I" is able to know its luminous being. The "I" in question is in the first place Yama as Lord of Death, for none can know the *Atman* who has not conquered death.

Secondly, it is the Higher Self of Nachiketas who has died to the outward life of sense and is now in the process of being reborn into the Higher Self as the spiritual son of the Teacher. Thirdly, it carries on the thought of verses 8 and 9 that the *Ātman* must be proclaimed by 'another.' Who is it then that is able to know the *Ātman* asks the Teacher. Only that Unknown 'Who' (*Ka*) who is *madanyo*, other-than-me, in other words the knowing principle that is beyond the limitations of self.[1]

Note also that the *Ātman* is said to rejoice and rejoice not, its indescribable bliss being beyond the opposites known to us as joy and sorrow. Like bodiless light it stands in the illuminated bodies, it changes not, nor moves, though all around is flux. Not all the elemental powers of the Universe can move it from its abiding place. Bodies may be shattered into tiny fragments by the force of high explosives, or may disintegrate in the grip of disease and death: worlds themselves may fly to pieces at the impact of some other heavenly body and yet the Life which ensouled those forms remains just where it was, where it will always be, the one fixed rock amid the tossing waste of waters.

He who would realise its being must fear no paradox, however strange, since the *Ātman* is the Unity out of which arise all the polar opposites that make up a world. Only by holding both the opposing poles firmly in view can we reach that which is both and neither. Everything we isolate or point out has its opposing counterglow, its reflection, or, as we say, its opposite. Therefore old pictures often represent the Initiate as standing with the Sun in one hand and the Moon in the other. With our right hands we must grasp the Sun and with

[1] Compare also the Vedik Unknown God, the God *Ka* or 'Who.'

our 'feminine' left hands the Moon. Then both must be brought together so that the Fire of the New Birth may leap forth as does the spark when flint is clashed with steel. Only so can we transcend the opposites of the mental vision and see anew in the all-unifying light of the *buddhi* beyond.

(23) *This* Ātman *is not to be attained by exposition, nor by intellectual thinking nor by much hearing (of traditional scripture). That* (Ātman) *indeed which he (the disciple) seeks, by that* (Ātman) *is it attained. To such a one the* Ātman *reveals its own form.*   .

This is a verse which is susceptible of more than one possible translation.

I have followed Shankara who comments *Yameva swātmānam esha sādhakovrinute prārthayate, tenaivātmānā varitrā swayamātma labhyo jñāyata evamityetat.*

Dualist commentators such as Madhva split up the sentence differently so as to read "he is to be attained only by him whom he chooses out. To such a one he reveals his own form." Thus they obtain a doctrine of Grace of which one can only say that it is conspicuous by its absence from all the other early Upanishads and reads very strangely in this context. Even Hume, the missionary translator, who is naturally predisposed to a rendering in accordance with theistic ways of thought, admits that "this doctrine of salvation through the Grace of the Creator is directly opposed to the general Upanishadic doctrine of salvation through knowledge." Moreover, if we look at the verse as a whole, we find it is not discussing the question of *who* can attain the *Ātman* but *by what means.* After enumerating various means by which it cannot be attained, it is natural for it to go on to state the means by which, rather than the person by whom, it can be attained. As

Shankara points out and as we have already stated earlier, the *Ātman* itself is its own means of attainment. As some of the alchemists remarked "without gold it is impossible to make gold," a saying that has caused considerable merriment among the learnedly ignorant. The truth is that nothing that is manifest, nothing that is 'apart' from the *Ātman*, can be a means to its attainment. "Nothing that is embodied, nothing that is conscious of separation, nothing that is out of the Eternal can aid you." In other words, nothing that is experienced in the mode of separateness, whether it be a human teacher or a sacred book, a 'yogic' exercise, or a magical ceremonial, can be a means to the attainment of the unitive mode of experience.

We are reminded of the interview between Bodhidharma and the exoterically devout Chinese Emperor. The latter asked how much merit he had acquired by the construction of a large number of temples and the translation of many sacred books. He was greatly offended when he was told "none at all." To the further question as to what was the most important of sacred doctrines, Bodhidharma replied: "Where all is Void, nothing can be called holy."

Shankara has also left a verse to the same effect:

"One may study Scriptures or sacrifice to Gods,
Perform all action or devote oneself to worship;
Without a realisation of the unity of the Atmān,
No liberation will be achieved even in a hundred
                                        Brāhmik Ages."[1]

Nothing that is conscious of separation, nothing that is thought of or felt as separate can be a means and to think that it can is to make a very great mistake. Nevertheless it would be an even greater mis-

---

[1] *Viveka Chuḍāmaṇi*, verse 6.

take to ignore teachers, teaching and practice altogether, for, in that case, at least for the overwhelming majority of aspirants, nothing whatever will result. True, neither teacher nor teaching, thought of as separate, can lead one to the Goal. But is there any need to think of them as separate? We have already seen that the Teacher is in truth the expression of the inner Teacher, the *Atman's* own Voice and if the disciple looks at Him in that Light he is far from useless.

Moreover in all experience,—and the entire universe from stars to electrons, from the Brahma-world to the grossest physical 'matter' *is* experience, nothing but experience—in all such there are two poles or modes. There is no separation without unity, and, in the manifest world at least, there is no unity without separation. Both modes are present in all experience and the whole question turns on which of them we are going to emphasise. The usefulness of the Teacher and teaching lies in their ability to direct our attention away from its habitual pre-occupation with the separateness and towards the unitive aspect which *is present all the time.*

Since it is just the unitive aspect that is the expression of the *Atmān*, which is in fact the light of the *Atman*, the meaning of our verse becomes quite clear. It is by the Light of the *Atman* that the *Atman* is seen. To him who cleaves to the unitive mode of experience, who sees the unitary aspect of all things, the transcendent Unity which is the *Atman* gradually reveals its true nature. Both Teachers and teaching can be of great help in assisting us to arrange our experience so that such seeing in the unitive mode becomes easier. In saying this we must not suppose that the doctrine of Grace which the later theistic commentators read into the verse is utterly without foundation. It is a dangerous, a two-edged doctrine, because it almost inevitably leads the aspirant to wait idly on the pleasure of a higher Power; in doing which he resembles the man, who, wishing to cross the Ganga, sat down by the bank waiting for it to finish flowing by. The doctrine is apt to strike at the very root of all effort, to lead to doctrines of special 'election' and in general to an anthropomorphic, sentimental and altogether dubious conception of the Power which, as Sri Krishna tells us, is "the same to all beings."[1]

Nevertheless there is a fact which we shall do well to remember, namely, that, as the Upanishad has told us several times, the Teaching, to be effective, must come from one who is *madanyaḥ*, other than 'myself.' This is natural, for the self is the very central focus of all separation and therefore, as we have seen, can be of no use to us in our quest. The Teaching must come from the Light beyond the mind and therefore be from a source other than self. Any idea that may come to the disciple, that 'I have attained thus far, I will attain further' will inevitably result in his falling back again into the sense of separateness. Hence, though we must disagree with any doctrine which attributes, or even tends to attribute, attainment to the 'favour' of a personal or quasi-personal deity, yet the stress laid on love and *bhakti* by the 'gracious' schools is a true one for the simple reason that loving as opposed to thinking is the great unitive mode. The separative mind must die and be transcended before we can pass beyond. The wings of love will carry us moth-like, straight through the dead-centre of self-hood to the Divine Flame beyond, the Flame that will consume all separateness.

But that love is not something that is bestowed on us by 'grace,' something for which we must simply wait in patience. Rather it is a mode of being

[1] Gita 9. 29.

that is present eternally in all beings whatsoever, something which is present in us like the flower in the plant and which will manifest at the right time, namely, when sufficient growth has taken place. Efforts will not cause it to blossom: that is quite true. Nevertheless the putting forth of the buds of effort by the disciple is a sign, a sure sign, that the blossoming will soon take place. True efforts, like true Faith, are an outward expression of inner knowledge, a knowledge that is none the less real because it is as yet hidden from the waking consciousness. "The Golden Flower is the Light, what colour has the Light? One uses the Golden Flower as an image. It is the true power of the transcendent Great One—The Great *One* is the term given to that which has nothing above it."[1] This passage from a Chinese book might have and, indeed, in a sense has come, from the same source as our Upanishad. Let us repeat: the Light of the *Ātman* is ever present in all experience; "the Light that shineth in darkness though the darkness comprehendeth it not." That Light must be attended to or 'picked out' as verse 13 put it. In proportion as we are able to pick it out it will become brighter. "Steadily as you watch and worship its Light will grow stronger." That Light itself is the Guide which leads us on the Way; it is also the Way itself and the final Goal into which, like the sea at the mouth of an estuary, the River of Life expands. Long ago as a tiny rivulet that River took its rise in the far-off snows. Its course has taken it through jungles, deserts and populous cities, but, all the time, it has been seeking the Sea in which alone it has its true being. Like calls to like; like has its home in like. It was the call of the Sea that was the motive power of the whole journey and it is to union with the Sea

---

[1] *The Secret of the Golden Flower.*

that it now so slowly and majestically glides. Yet never in the whole long journey has it been one hair's breadth outside its Home. From the *Ātman,* in the *Ātman,* to the *Ātman* has been the pilgrimage of the Soul, for, in the realm of spirit, Height is the same as Depth, the Snowy Peak one with the Sea's Abyss.

(24) *Not he who has not detached himself from evil conduct, not he (whose senses) are not tranquil, not he whose (psyche) is not unified, not he whose mind is not at peace can attain this* (Ātman) *by any knowing.*

The previous verse having dealt with the means by which the knowledge of the *Ātman* can and cannot be gained, the present one goes on to state certain obstacles, and by implication, certain essential qualifications that the aspirant must have.

In the first place, the search is useless unless the disciple has definitely turned away from bad conduct. This is no question of "if you aren't a good boy I shan't give you any sweets," no mere infringement of a moral code, no mere offence against a personal God, but a statement based on definite philosophical principles. 'Bad' or 'evil' conduct is action (in thought and feeling as well as in deeds) which increases the sense of separateness. In the last analysis all 'evil' conduct reduces itself to this. To injure another is 'evil' because it springs from, and consequently intensifies, the false notion that that 'other' is something separate from 'me,' something whose injury may benefit and cannot possibly harm me. Even self-injury or suicide, often enough performed out of pique and with the idea either that 'it doesn't matter what happens to me' or that 'I shall make so and so sorry he ever spoke to me like that'; even such comes in the same category for, even in the former alternative, it

ignores the fact that 'I' am not separate from the whole,
and that, if I injure myself, I injure the whole.

The above principle serves as a negative test
also. That which does not increase the sense of separateness is not 'evil', whatever the moral codes may say.
Nevertheless it is always wise to pause before deciding
to flout established moral codes; for the latter often
embody age-old wisdom, and, so long as *desire* for separateness lurks in our hearts, it is only too easy for us to
deceive ourselves with plausible reasonings. Certainly
the disciple has to learn to dispense with the aid of
artificial traffic-lights but before he can do so safely he
must have pretty thoroughly mastered the vehicle
which he is driving.

In any case it is entirely certain and even self-
evident that he who acts or thinks in such way as to
increase the sense of separateness cannot possibly, as
long as he does so, attain to the seeing of the *Átman*
which depends upon the other, the unitive mode, of
experiencing.

"He whose senses are not tranquil." We have
already shown how the senses are the sails by which
the winds of desire carry off the ship of the Soul.
If they are not at rest it is quite impossible to gain
the Knowledge for they will constantly carry the
psyche outwards into external objects and so prevent it
from plunging into the central Well in which the *Átman*
dwells. This verse being merely a preliminary and
negative statement, we shall say nothing here about the
method by which the senses are to be tranquillised.

The next statement is that the Knowledge cannot
be gained by one who is not *samāhita*, a word which
means held together, combined, unified. It is often
taken as meaning concentrated in meditation but in
truth that is covered in the next statement, and this
is a wider one, a pre-requisite of any successful medi-

113

8

tation. In most men there is serious disunion between the two sides of their natures that we term the thinking and feeling sides respectively. In some the faculty of thought is overvalued and developed at the expense of feeling, and, in others, the opposite. But the psyche is a unity and any over-emphasis on one side means that the other will be stunted, underdeveloped and consequently out of harmony with the more developed side. It will moreover be filled with feelings of revenge against the dominating power which keeps it in the dark and thus there will be a state of war, sometimes open, more often latent, within the dwelling of the Soul. The feeling-self, (if that be the inferior side), like a subject people, will take delight in secretly thwarting the purposes of the dominant thinking mind, even though, in the process, itself is injured too. Within us are the Sun and Moon and if these are not in harmonious aspect with each other, if, as astrologers say, they are 'in square,' a state of inner conflict is inevitable. "A house that is divided against itself cannot stand": there can be no harmony within the psyche unless the Sun of thought and the Moon of feeling are equally valued and consequently equally developed. Only then will the Sacred Marriage be possible and the Divine Birth, the birth of Knowledge take place.

In the outer world too the same disharmony is found. The subjection of woman which has characterised most of the dominant sections of mankind is responsible for the present chaotic state of world affairs, both for the indolent 'backwardness' of the East and the active *Āsurik* evil of the West.[1] This

---

[1] Note the 'happiness' which so many have remarked in the Burmese people. It is no coincidence that, among these happy people, women enjoy more freedom of status than almost anywhere else in the world.

has been very generally realised in recent years but what is not so widely understood is that its real cause is to be found in the overvaluation of the male thinking function (on the part of those, at least, who come to the top and stand at the helm of the destinies of nations) and the consequent under-valuation of the 'female' function of feeling. Small wonder is it that when the feeling mode does succeed in breaking out—the leader of the Nazis has said more than once that he thinks with his 'blood' rather than with his head—it should do so in a catastrophic form which threatens to destroy all that the thinking mind has so carefully built up through centuries of toil.

We have digressed into outer affairs in order to give a more vivid idea of the state in which the average and disunited psyche actually is, a state of horrible and cataclysmic war. That this is so is entirely certain since the war which is now raging in Europe is only the outer projection of the inner psychic condition and nations get, not only the governments, but the wars that they deserve. With this we will leave the outer and return to the inner world with which we are concerned. In that inner world it is absolutely certain that he whose psyche is not harmoniously unified will never enter the *Atman's* kingdom of Heaven. Perhaps that was one reason why Christ told his followers that they must become as little children, for in such the inner disharmony which afflicts most grown men has not had time to develop, and, as Wordsworth said, "Heaven lies about us in our infancy." Old age is indeed a second childhood and death a second birth, but that second childhood is for most of us one which is seamed with the follies and strife of adult life. Only in the mystic Childhood and the mystic Death is there that serene harmony which even ordinary childhood symbolises rather than actually possesses.

The peace of mind which is the next to be mentioned can never be gained until the psyche is *samāhita* or
harmoniously united. Many pass years in fruitless attempts to calm their minds and bring them to rest in
'meditation' and often in the end have to give up the
effort in despair, crying out, like Arjuna, "O Madhu-
sūdana, I see no stable foundation for this Yoga on
account of the restlessness of the mind."[1] My mind
is so unstable: how can I learn to concentrate it?
These are the questions which again and again we
put to those whom we have reason to suppose have
travelled further than ourselves on this Path. We
do not realise that the master is held in bondage by his
own slave and that as long as we continue to suppress
one side of our psyche there can be no meditation for us.
Feeling, become hostile through subjection, thwarts
in a thousand lurking ambushes the proud determination of our minds. We can concentrate quite efficiently
when our feelings are sympathetically aroused. Does
not a lover concentrate on his beloved, a business man
on his beloved accounts? When, however, we seek
to concentrate our minds in Yoga, our feelings suddenly
thwart us and a thousand desire-born images and fancies
invade our minds just when we want to still them.

Here again we see why *Bhakti* is so important, not
as a separate path of its own, but as one side of the one
Path which all must tread. Until there is inner psychic
unity, there will be no concentration of mind. As Sri
Krishna teaches—"There is no intuitive knowledge
(*buddhi*) for the non-harmonised, nor for the non-
harmonised is there concentration. For him without concentration there is no peace and for the un-
peaceful, where is happiness."[2] First we must abs-

[1] Gita 6. 33.
[2] Gita 2. 66.

tain from action which increases separateness. Secondly, we must tranquillise our senses. Thirdly, we must harmonise the opposing forces in our selves. Then and only then shall we be able to meditate in peace, then and only then will the Knowledge manifest in our hearts. Till then, no process of knowing will lead us where we have to go, beyond the mental vision which sees the world as the arena of endless strife between the opposites.

Note, however, that the text does not say that these are the means of Knowledge. The Knowledge is eternally existent, as the previous verse told us, and there are no means to it except itself. By the *Atman's* Light is the *Atman* seen. The conditions in this verse are only the indispensable prerequisites. As long as they are not acquired, there can be no knowledge of the unitive Light. Nevertheless the Light is ever present, even in the darkness, and, once more, "When the disciple is ready, the Guru will appear."

(25) *He for whom the Brāhman and the Kshattriya are both food and for whom Death is but a sauce—who can thus know where He is.*

The section ends with this somewhat cryptic verse. The Brāhman and Kshattriya, the two dominant castes, represent the two aspects of the mind, the first, the mind turned inward in contemplation thus serving as the intermediary between Gods and men, and the second, that mind turned outwards towards action and thus serving as the ruler and fighter. These are the two poles of the mind and therefore both are said to be as food, i.e., substance for the Unitary *Atman* beyond. Death, too, is but a change-over from the outgoing to the ingoing mode and is thus said to be an 'oversprinkling,' a sort of sauce that is added, as we might say, to give variety. Change, as an old proverb has it, is the spice of life and the change we know as death is the tidal ebb and flow which keeps sweet the waters of the great Sea.

Who can in truth know where to find that mystic Unity? Once more the answer, implied though not stated in the text, must be, 'Not-I.'

CHAPTER III

We have already seen in the preceding sections that the crux of the whole is the nature of self. By self we are bound in the ignorance and in Self we find the Knowledge. This third section, therefore, takes up the whole question of the nature of man and the various levels or principles of his being.

(1) *There are two that partake of the Cosmic Order in the World of good deeds. Both have entered into the secret Cave (of the heart) in the superior, the upper worlds of being. Those who know the Secret Teachings (Brahmavidaḥ) and those Five-Fired ones who have kindled the triple Nachiketas Fire, know them as Light and Shade.*

The Universe or Cosmic Egg is divided into two halves, an upper and a lower, between which stand the *mānasik* points, the Individual egos. The Upper Half is reflected in and as the Lower Half, each individual ego being, so to speak, the focal centre through which this reflection takes place. Sometimes these two Halves have been referred to as Spirit and Matter and symbolised by the well known symbol of the interlaced triangles with the central point. Sometimes again the symbol has been varied and we get the triangles placed point to point, giving us the *Ḍamaru* or double drum of Shiva, the *Kamaṇḍalu* of Brahmā, the Hour-Glass of Saturn, and the sacred double-headed axe of the Cretan mysteries. The Upper Hemisphere has also been spoken of as the *Mons Philosophorum*, the Mountain of the Philosophers, symbolised in India by Mount Meru, also Mount Kailash.

In truth, however, we must only apply the terms Spirit and Matter to these Cosmic Hemispheres with caution, for Spirit and Matter represent the two ultimate Poles of being. In themselves they are beyond all that is strictly manifest, beyond, that is, the Brahma-world or Cosmic Egg. All that is contained within that Egg is formed of their interplay and consequently it is only in the sense of predominant manifestation that we can speak of the Upper Hemisphere as Spirit, the lower as Matter.

Each of them is triply divided (the three points of the triangles) and the upper trinity is reflected, though in an inverted manner, in the lower. As the Kabala teaches, *Demon est Deus inversus*, the Devil is the inverted reflection of God.

The two trinities with the central focal point make up the well-known Seven Worlds, the seven modes of manifested being, known in Indian teaching as *Bhūr, Bhuvas, Swar, Mahas, Jana, Tapas, Satya*.

We may also note in passing that these two Hemispheres have their reflections down here on this physical plane, though, in the process, the vertical has become horizontal, $\underline{\mathbf{X}}$ has become $\bowtie$. Thus we have the right and left hemisphere of the brain, controlling the left and right hands respectively, a fact upon which we will not enlarge, though it is full of intense significance for those who can see. Again we have the Eastern and Western hemispheres of the earth, another fact of great meaning in spite of all that spherical geometry may have to say about the relativity of all such divisions. Whatever difficulties geographers may feel in drawing the dividing lines, the difference of East and West is a fact of profound psychic importance. Notwithstanding all the cheap sneers of the ignorant, East and West *do* stand for, and are the homes of 'Spirit' and 'Matter' respectively—at least in the present precessional cycle.

However, we will not pursue these secondary manifestations or reflections any further but will keep to our main theme, the 'vertical' division of the manifested universe into the two great hemispheres, composed respectively of the three worlds of 'Spirit' and the three of 'Matter.' Those who prefer so-called philosophical terms may substitute for the above the more cumbersome and no more accurate words, subjectivity and objectivity. In the Vedas they are known as *Dhyāvāprithivī*, Heaven and Earth, the Universal Parents.

We need not concern ourselves here with the details of the Seven Worlds, for all that the text deals with is the division into the two Hemispheres, in one of which, the upper, subjective, spiritual or Heavenly, dwell the Two. Who or what are these two ? In another Upanishad we meet them again as "two Birds, fast friends, dwelling in the one Tree,"[1] and in the Gita they are referred to as the two Purushas, the *kshara* or perishable and the *akshara* or imperishable.[2] They are in fact the Heavenly Twins, the two selves, and, like other symbols, they have more than one meaning, or rather, may be applied to more than one octave of being.

In the first place we may take Light as referring to the ordinary personal ego of waking consciousness, in which case Shade is our 'inferior self,' those parts of the psyche to which we do not care to direct our attention, whose existence we do not care to admit and which are consequently what psychologists term 're-pressed'. Jung, indeed, has somewhere referred to

1 *Muṇḍaka Upanishad* 3. 1. 1.
2 *Gita* 15. 16.

this hidden and inferior self as the shadow. We may add that, though its existence is not usually admitted by ourselves, it is often painfully evident to others in our actions. When confronted by its manifestations people are apt to say of us that we "have a very unpleasant side to our nature sometimes" or again that we "weren't ourselves that day" or "have got out of bed on the wrong side."

This, however, is not the scale with which our text is concerned, so that, though it is a subject of great interest and importance, we will pass on, having only mentioned it for the sake of completeness.

On a higher scale we may take them as the personal and individual selves respectively and this, indeed, is the first form in which we meet them. Light is thus the permanent focus, the Higher or individual Ego, that which endures on its own plane of being throughout the aeons of cosmic duration, sending forth shadow after shadow, the transient personal selves that manifest in our world of birth and death. On this scale the shadow is the empirical self of waking life, our conscious personality, the ignorant and petty self of daily life, a self which comes into being at, or rather shortly after, birth and which disintegrates sometime after bodily death, its garnered experience, or such of it as is of any value, returning to the Light which sent it forth.

This again is not the scale to which our text primarily refers since in this case both Light and Shade are said to dwell in the upper Hemisphere and this can scarcely be said of the ordinary waking personal self except in the case of an aspirant whose lower self has even now united with the Higher. Such a one is indeed Nachiketas but the statement in the text seems to have a wider application.

Hence we have here to take them in a still higher

sense, the sense of *Mahat-buddhi*. These two, referred
to in verse 13 as the Great Self and the Self of Knowledge, are the two great moments of the Great Brahma-
world or world of *Mahat* taken as one whole. We shall
have to refer to them again later (chapter 6 verse 5) but
may anticipate a little here. In the Vedik hymns they
are known as the dual *Mitra-Varuna, Mitra,* Lord of the
Day Sky and *Varuna,* Lord of the Night Sky. As
Day and Night they are the two halves of the great
circle of Brāhmik being. Themselves the first manifestations of the Unmanifest Pair beyond,[1] they are
the archetypal Parents of all lesser dualities in the
worlds below, including of course the duality of the
higher and lower minds. Hence they are pre-eminently
the Two who partake of the *rita* or Cosmic Order
which is the totality of the Brahma-world, the world
in which the entire manifested cosmos exists as one harmonious whole.

Of the two, Light is *Mahat*, the radiant and creative
Sun, the manifest projection of the hidden *Shānta Ātman*,
while Shade is *Buddhi*, the cool Goddess of the Night,
Bride of the Sun and daughter of the *Mūla-prakriti* beyond.[2] Hence the Moon is Wisdom's Daughter, the
manifest Body of the transcendent Wisdom itself and
when Cornelius Agrippa wrote that "in these twenty
eight (Lunar) mansions do lie hid many secrets of the

[1] i.e., the *Shānta Ātman* and the *Avyakta* or *Mūla-prakriti.*

[2] We should remember that 'shade' in a hot country has
somewhat different connotations from those it has in a cold one.
In India it suggests the cool shelter of the home and of the waters,
the rest of night after the heat of day, the sheltering arms of the
Mother, the cool draught of immortality. Buddhist books are full
of praises of the 'coolness' of the saving Wisdom, the Bodhi
(=buddhi), and, as Coomaraswami has pointed out, the Rigveda
speaks of going to Agni (who of course is dual) "as to the shade
from fervent heat." R. V. VI. 16. 38.

wisdom of the Ancients, by which they wrought wonders on all things which are under the circle of the Moon" his words bore a far deeper meaning than that of ordinary astrology and phenomenal magic. He who knows in its fulness the Course of the Moon has mastered the Wisdom.

Just as the sun and moon circle above us in the heavens, weaving between them the harmonies of day and night, summer and winter, so do the Two circle above us, as the text says, in the superior Worlds of Being, weaving the mighty web of the Cosmic Harmony. Truly do the knowers of Brahman speak of Them as Light and Shade for it is by the contemplation of the mysteries of light and shade here below that we too can become knowers of Brahma. He who knows Light and Shade, and their interaction (which is how we perceive their unity), knows the whole Universe with all that is in it. He knows not only that *demon est deus inversus*, but, as Nāgarjuna even more profoundly stated it, that "*Nirvāna* and *Samsāra* are the same." He has achieved the Harmony, and, new-born of the two Divine Parents, he manifests in himself as Third or Son, the divine *Rita* which is eternally partaken[1] of by the Two above. Now is he in truth reborn by the New Birth from, as Hermes puts it, "Wisdom that understands in Silence (Shade) and the True Good (Light)." In the phrase of the Orphic Initiate he is "a Son of Earth and Starry Heaven," in that of the Christian, "very God and very Man."[2]

---

[1] Notice that the word *pibantau* literally means 'drinking,' a clear reference to the cool draught of the Elixir of Life.

[2] The Naasene document, speaking of the souls who are re-born by this Divine Birth says:—"They passed by the Streams of Ocean (*Varuṇa*) and by the White Rocks (*Mitra*), the Gates of the Sun (*Light*), and the People of Dreams (*Shade*). For Ocean is birth-causing of Gods and birth-causing of men, flowing

Chapter III

As for the Two Divine Ones, the Parents, they are to be sought for, as the text suggests, in the Secret Cave of the Heart because there in the mystic Centre and there alone are they to be found. To look for them in the disharmony and separation of the outer and lower worlds is mere waste of time and effort.

We must pause for a moment, however, over the phrase 'the world of good deeds' '*Sukritasya loke*,' a phrase which, like so many others, has two meanings. From one point of view the reference is to the Worlds that are enjoyed after death, the state in which the Individual Self enjoys, in what the Gita calls "the wide-extended heaven world", the fruits of its good deeds. Good deeds, as we have seen, mean harmonious deeds, and, after the death of the body, the self enjoys such portions of the Great Harmony as its deeds down here have placed it in touch with, enjoys them in a state that is *to us* subjective or dream-like but which is perfectly objective to him who enjoys it and is, indeed, the Heaven of exoteric religion. As for the Divine Self, that, of course, exists and partakes for ever in the Harmony.

Underneath this meaning, however, is another. The Secret Teachings, as opposed to those of exoteric religions, are never about matters which can only be experienced after death but are intended for realisation here and now. From this point of view '*loka*' (world or plane of being) means, as both Shankara and Madhva point out, this human body which has been gained as the result of previous good deeds.[1] It is within this body, in its

---

and ebbing for ever, now up and now down. When Ocean flows down it is birth-causing of men; and when up towards the Wall and Palisade (the *uppermost limit of manifestation*) and the White Rocks (*the heavenly Sun*) it is birth-causing of Gods." G. R. S. Mead's translation: italics mine.

[1] We need not interpret this in the sense of the popular notion that one human birth may be sandwiched in between many

very heart and inmost recesses, that the Two are to be sought for and found. As Paracelsus expressed it: "Whoever desires to be a practical philosopher ought to be able to indicate heaven and hell in the microcosm, the little universe, and to find everything in man that exists in heaven or on earth."

The phrase *Brahma-vidaḥ*, which we have translated as the knowers of the Secret Teachings, means literally he who knows the One Reality, the *Brahman*. Nevertheless, as the word *Brahma* also means the sacred mantras, we have preferred the above rendering as more suitable in the present context.

The Five-Fired ones are those who maintain the five sacrificial fires, the householders as opposed to the ascetics or presumptive Brahma-knowers. In reality the Five Fires are the five great Cosmic Elemental Fires which burn on the five manifested levels of the universe and which are reflected in this world in the form of the fires of the five senses. Those senses are, like all fires, good servants but bad masters, and it is the duty of the disciple to see that they burn, not all over the place, but controlled on sacrificial altars on which are offered the various objects of sense.

"Some offer sound and the other four sense objects as sacrifice in the fires of the senses."[1] All who live have the Five Fires but only those who know the Sacred Hidden Fire, the triple Nachiketas Fire, are able to transmute the offerings and make of them a means of ascent to the Enduring. Hence it is to this Sacred Fire that the teaching returns.

---

births in the form of animals. What is meant is that our present status as self-conscious, thinking beings is the result of ages of evolution, an evolution that was helped on by 'good' deeds and hindered by 'evil' ones.

[1] Gita 4-26.

Chapter III

(2) We are able to master that Nachiketas Fire which is the Bridge of those who sacrifice, and which (leads to)[1] the highest imperishable Brahman, the fearless Other Shore for those who wish to cross.

The Nachiketas Fire is the central secret of this Upanishad. Inadequate stress has been laid upon it by most translators who have probably felt that it was only one of the ritualistic fires that ancient India used to believe in. Consequently, many of them have translated differently so as to separate the Fire, which, according to them, is only the Bridge which leads to Heaven or the Brahma world, from the Supreme Imperishable *Brahma*, attainable only by Knowledge. If this were true, however, there would be absolutely no point in Yama's recurring to the Sacred Fire at this particular juncture.

It is true that as we have already seen, nothing that is non-eternal can be a means to the Eternal,[2] but it is also true that It is not to be attained by 'exposition' (*pravachana*) either, nor as shown in chapter II, verse 24, will any mode of knowing suffice for him who has not thoroughly transmuted his whole being. Mere ritual fires will no doubt be useless for this purpose but the Nachiketas Fire is not a mere ritual fire but the secret alchemical Fire which is the means of transmutation. It therefore is the Bridge which leads to the Great Being of the Brahma-world and it is from that world that, on the path of gradual liberation, the final and unaided flight is made, the flight of the alone to the Alone. Not only is the Fire, the Bridge which leads

---

[1] Not only "leads to"; in an important sense the Fire *is* the Supreme *Brahman* which is what the text itself reads if taken literally as it stands.

[2] *Kaṭha* 2. 10.

to the Brahman.   As indicated in a previous foot-note, in a very important sense it is itself the *Parabrahman*, the One unmanifest but Living Power which is that *Parabrahman's* very Heart.   Such statements, however, are impossible to understand with the mind and it is easier to conceive it as the Power which manifests in the Cosmos. In itself, however, it is that most mysterious of all Fires, the hidden Black Fire mentioned in the Zohar—the fire of which all the various coloured fires are manifestations.

Those who wish to interpret this Upanishad as solely concerned with the path of Sudden Liberation must do so, though, as in the case of the Gita, they will have to strain the text.   For the rest, explanations and expositions can not give the Knowledge for which transmutation is necessary and transmutation can only be achieved by the Nachiketas Fire.   Mere metaphysical explanations are but a painted flame, a thing as useless as a still-born child.   Only the True Fire can serve as the Bridge, and, even then, that Bridge is one whose arches crumble to dust behind the leaping feet.

"On either hand as far as eye could see,
A great black swamp and of an evil smell,
Part black, part whitened with the bones of men,
Not to be crost, save that some ancient king
Had built a way, where, linked with many a
bridge,
A thousand piers ran into the great Sea.
And Galahad fled along them bridge by bridge,
And every bridge as quickly as he crost
Sprang into fire and vanished, tho' I yearned to
follow."[1]

The secret of the Fire must be known if we would

[1] Tennyson's *Holy Grail*.

cross the dark and evil swamp. Without it, mere intellectual study, whether dignified by the title Vedānta or by any other such name, is but the building of a mental tower of Babel, an aspiration to a Heaven that no bricks of words or thought can ever reach, a thing whose useless ruins remain to view as one more 'Philosopher's Folly.'

How many are there not who spend whole life times in the study of Vedānta and kindred philosophies and yet who have to confess to themselves in the end that nothing has happened. The world has remained the same world, their senses have remained the same vicious and unruly horses, the Light that was to have shone forth has remained hidden and the Unitive Knowledge of which they have read and argued so much has remained a metaphysical theory, something the experience of which must be postponed till after death.

All this is through ignorance of the Fire, which, as the verse tells us, is the Bridge for those who sacrifice: these last, by the way, not being those who offer the exoteric and ritualistic offerings, but those who tread the inner Path of Sacrifice. It is the indispensable Bridge for those who would in very truth make the Journey. As we have quoted before "one must not wish to leave out the steps between and penetrate directly." Only across this Bridge can we travel from Earth to Heaven, from Death to Immortality.

The Secret Fire is the Fire which burns in the heart of the Sun, in the heart of man and in the heart of the World. Like a great Rose of Light it burns for ever, "Rose of all Roses, Rose of all the World": its eight flame-petals sound forth in silence the one Great Sound. He who can bathe naked in its Flame has won Immortality. It is the Wondrous Flame that Arjuna saw, a sacrificial Fire whose splendour consumed the

Worlds.[1]

It is also the *Vaishwānara*, the Fire of Life, which, seated in the bodies of all living beings, united with the life-breath, transmutes the four kinds of food, i.e., the other four elements.[2]

These too are the Rose leaves by the eating of which the candidate for initiation transmuted his animal form into the "human form divine."[3] It was of this Fire that Heracleitus wrote: "This world order, the same for all beings, neither any of the gods hath made nor any man; but it was always, is and shall be ever-living Fire, kindled in measure and quenched in measure."[4] The Veda, and indeed all mystical literature, is saturated with it. We shall only make one further quotation, one which is perhaps less widely known. In an old Rosicrucian manuscript it is written:

"Strive for the fire,
Seek the fire:
So thou wilt find the fire.
Light a fire.
Put fire to fire.
Boil fire in fire.
Throw body soul and spirit into fire,
So shalt thou get dead and living fire,
Out of which will come black, yellow, white and
red fire,
Bear thy Children in fire,
Feed, give them to drink, nourish them in fire,[5]

---

[1] Gita Chapter XI, Verse 19, and others.
[2] Gita 15. 14.
[3] Apuleius. *The Golden Ass.*
[4] Heracleitus Fragment D. 30.
[5] Remember the Fire in which Demeter, Goddess of the Eleusinian Mysteries, bathed the child of her host to render it immortal.

So will they live and die in fire,
And be fire and stay in fire.
Their silver and gold will become fire,
Heaven and Earth will perish in fire,
And become finally a philosopher's fire."

And again:

"Whoever seeks it, suffer.
Whoever finds it, be silent.
Whoever holds it, hide it,
Whoever may use it, do so unbeknown.
Whoever is a true Philosopher,
Remain nameless,
Trust no one but God.
For loyalty flew from earth heavenwards and left all men whose mind is upon earthly matter."[1]

(3) *Know the* Ātman *as Lord of the Chariot, the body as the Chariot itself: know the* buddhi *to be the Charioteer and the mind* (manas) *as the reins.*

(4) *The senses, they say, are the Horses, the sense-objects the path on which they run. The* Ātman *united to senses and mind is said by the wise to be the Experiencer* (bhoktā).

(5) *He who is without intuitive judgement*[2] *and whose*

---

[1] *Secret Symbols of the Rosicrucians.*

[2] The word used is *Vijñāna*, a synonym of *buddhi*. It may also be loosely translated as wisdom. Compare Gita IX. 1. where *Jñāna* and *Vijñāna* have, according to Sridhara, the significance of Knowledge and Experience respectively. We may also note the *Vijñānamaya purusha* of the *Taittirīya Upanishad* which is equivalent to *buddhi*. Perhaps discriminative knowledge would be a good rendering if it did not suggest the separative analytic discrimination of *manas* whereas here the discrimination is the power of referring the given act or event to the pattern of the whole.

mind (manas) *is not constantly controlled, his senses become unmanageable like the vicious horses of a charioteer.*

(6) *But he who has intuitive judgement, whose mind is ever held firm, his senses are controllable like the good horses of a charioteer.*

(7) *He who is without intuitive judgement and is of un-controlled mind, ever impure, he does not reach that goal, but wanders in the Ocean of the World.*

(8) *But he who has intuitive judgement and is of con-trolled mind, ever pure, he attains that Goal* (padam) *whence he is born no more.*

(9) *The man who has intuitive judgement as his Charioteer and the mind as reins, gains the End of the Road. That is the Supreme abode of All-pervading Spirit* (Vishṇu).

Having set forth the means by which the Path is to be travelled, namely, the Sacred Fire, the Teacher goes on to explain the nature of the Path itself, that Path which starts from the heart of the disciple and of which it has been said "Thou canst not travel on the Path before thou hast become that Path itself."[1] The teaching that follows is for him who knows the Fire; for others, though they may seem to understand it, it will be of little avail; they will remain stuck fast in the bog of intellectual conceptions and no actual travel-ling, no transmutation, will take place. Subject to that reservation, the exposition is clear and simple enough. It is, however, as if one said wash the rice, place it in a pot and boil it till it is cooked—very simple, provided the would-be cook knows how to light the fire, but not much use if he does not.

In the first place the ancient symbol of the chariot is brought forward as representing the entire psycho-

[1] *Voice of the Silence.*

physical being that we call man. The body itself is said to be the chariot drawn by the horses of the senses. Those horses are controlled by the reins of *manas* held in the hands of *buddhi* the Driver. The *Ātman* itself is the Lord of the Chariot, he who sits quietly within it. The world of sense-objects is of course the road on which the chariot travels.

In this enumeration, body and senses call for no comment except the one that the senses are in reality twofold, outer and inner. The inner perceptions that we call sensuous imaginations or phantasies are as much Horses as are those which we refer to the outer or physical world. Both sets of Horses, if not controlled, carry away the Chariot in a furious gallop, and, of the two, the inner senses are the more dangerous. The Gītā warns us of the danger of controlling the outer while allowing the inner a free rein.[1]

Before going any further we may note the universality of this chariot symbolism. The Kabala has much to say about the Mercabah or Sacred Chariot (which is depicted on one of the Tarot Trumps) and Philo, the Alexandrian Jew, writes of it in almost identical terms with our text, save that he is writing of the Universal or Macrocosmic chariot rather than of the microcosmic one. "So that he who drives the chariot of the Powers is the Logos and He who is borne in the chariot is He who speaks (the Logos) giving commandment to the Driver for the right driving of the universe."[2]

Plato uses this symbol and applies it in the same microcosmic sense as does our text. He describes the horses of the Soul's Chariot as being a pair, one noble and the other ignoble, and says that "as might be ex-

[1] Gita 3. 6.
[2] Translated by G. R. S. Mead in *Thrice Greatest Hermes*, I, 238.

pected, there is a great deal of trouble in managing them."

"Of the Souls whosoever followeth God best and is being made most like unto Him, keepeth the Head of her Charioteer lifted up in the space without the firmament (the inner space of the Divine World), so she is carried round with the circuit thereof, yet being still troubled with the Horses, and hardly beholding the Things-which-are; so she is now lifted up, now sinketh down, and, because of the compulsion of the Horses, seeth some of the Things-which-are, and some she seeth not."

"And the rest of the Souls (i.e., the inferior ones) you must know, follow, all striving after that which is above, but unable to reach it, and so are carried round together and sink under water, trampling upon one another, and running against one another, and pressing on for to outstrip one another with a mighty great sound of tumult and sweat."

"And here, by reason of the unskilfulness of the charioteers, many Souls are maimed and many have many feathers of their (horse's) wings broken, and all greatly travailing, depart without initiation in the Vision of That-which-is, and departing, betake them to the food of Opinion."[1]

We may note also the Gita, the whole teaching of which is set against a background of Chariot symbolism.

Returning to our text, we have seen that the body is the Chariot, the senses (outer and inner) the Horses and the sense-objects the paths they travel. Those Horses are to be controlled by the Driver, *buddhi* by the aid of the reins of *manas*, the Lord or rider in the Chariot being the *Ātman*, the Light of the One Self which per-

[1] Plato *Phaedrus*, Stewart's translation quoted by G. R. S. Mead, op. cit.

vades all things. These terms *ātmā*, *buddhi* and *manas* are, like so many others, capable of application on several scales and so in several apparent senses. This fluidity of application is a fact which must be borne in mind throughout, as, otherwise, if we become en-meshed in the one-word-one-application fallacy, nothing but confusion will result. Consequently we shall de-fine these terms in their most general sense and then show how they can be variously applied.

To start with *Ātmā*: it is the Light of consciring (or consciousness, to use the more familiar though less apt term), the ultimate principle of living Self-hood on any scale or level of being. In its most ultimate sense it is the one Spirit, the Light of the Worlds, what the Gita terms the *Kshetrajña* or Knower of the Field. It pervades all levels and all scales of being and thus is the ultimate Self of any unit, whether that unit be a universe, a world, a man, or an atom, for it is the Light which sustains all those patterns in existence and in which they have their being. It is important to realise that it is as much present in man's physical body (or even in a stone, for that matter) as in the depths of the Soul or of a God.

Manas and *buddhi* are the two powers of that Light, the former the power of seeing things as separate (and so of bringing about their apparent separation) and the latter of seeing things as a unity, all being related to all. Thus, when we perceive things as so many separate en-tities or events, as in scientific studies or in ordinary common-sense, that is the *mānasik* mode. When on the other hand, we see that:

> Nothing in the world is single,
> All things by a law divine,
> In one another's being mingle—[1]

[1] Shelley. *Love's Philosophy.*

the vision, in fact, of the mystic and the poet, we are seeing in the mode of the *buddhi*.

If a clear grasp of these two modes of consciring or 'seeing' is attained it becomes possible to pick out the elements of *manas* and *buddhi* respectively in any pattern of experience on any scale whatsoever. Without it we are lost at once. *Manas* becomes just that vague and blessed entity, 'the mind' and *buddhi* some sort of super-mind 'up beyond.' Thus we are back in the sterility of exoteric teaching in which all important things are postponed till 'after death.' In the esoteric teaching, on the other hand, everything that is, is *here and now*, and we must learn to pick it out of the matrix of our present experience. Only when we have done so does it become possible for that experience to expand into something wider and vaster.

Here and now, then, *Atmā* is the Light of Consciring, "the master light of all our seeing," *buddhi* the seeing of unity in experience, and *manas* the seeing of separateness and individualism.

We can thus see that what we know as the ego, whether the personal ego of daily life (sometimes called lower *manas*) or the individual and enduring Ego (higher *manas*), is essentially a manifestation of *manas*. On the other hand, the spirit which is beyond the ego and which sees all things as related and united to each other is, on any scale, a manifestation of *buddhi*.

For instance, in ordinary life, *manas* is present as the ego consciousness which says I, I, I; I am separate from you, I want, I wish and I will. Even while saying it, however, we are or can be aware of a still small voice which we call the voice of conscience, one which, saying 'not you but all', warns us of the selfishness of our thought. That voice which has in some schools been called the *antaḥkaraṇa*,[1] is in reality the Bridge which leads from the lower to the higher Self, i.e., from Shade to Light. But, just as we saw that Shade and Light were found on several scales, so is this Voice. It may be the Bridge between the personal and individual selves, or between that higher enduring Ego and the One Self of all beyond. In all cases, however, it is a manifestation of the principle of *buddhi*. In the Gita, for instance, we have *two* Charioteers, Sri Krishna himself being the charioteer of Arjuna, the enduring higher Ego and Sañjaya, Charioteer of *Dhritarāshtra*, the lower or personal self.[2] Both these are manifestations of the same principle but on different scales. It is important to realise this as they may or may not be given different names to suit the requirements of a particular teaching. In the most general sense we may say that that which makes two out of one is *manas*, that which makes one out of two is *buddhi*. Analysis is *mānasik*, synthesis *buddhik*.

The *buddhi*, then, is the vision which sees the pattern of the whole, and which, therefore, being able to take account of the whole, is pre-eminently the charioteer of the psyche. When the chariot is driven according to the dictates of the *buddhi*, no harm can ever come to it, for it will be driven in the spirit of the Cosmic Harmony in which there are and can be no mishaps. No man's chariot ever came to grief through following either the voice of conscience (provided it really was that voice) or the voice of the Spirit which is beyond all self. There is a famous Greek statue called the bronze charioteer. Straight and austerely fall the folds of his garments but they have a beauty that is far beyond all

---

[1] See the *Voice of the Silence*. In classic Vedānta, however, *antaḥkaraṇa* has a different significance.

[2] See my *Yoga of the Bhagavat Gita*—Prolegomena, p. xxiii.

the exuberant and flowing curves of sense, and the eyes gaze with a steady vision that pierces beyond the separateness of earthly forms to the eternal unity of the stars, a vision of what Plato termed the Things-which-are. None whose Horses are controlled by him will sink under the waters, nor trample on, nor run against, his fellows.

But even this Divine Charioteer needs reins with which to control the Horses. Those reins are furnished by the principle of *manas*. The disparity between the spiritual principle of *Buddhi*, the Dweller in the Upper Hemisphere of being, and the Horses of sense, the Dwellers in the lower half, is too great for the former to act directly on the latter. There was a time, indeed, when the lower Hemisphere truly reflected the Upper and when all was one Harmony. That, however, was many, many ages ago in that Golden Age which modern Europe and its apes have thought a fable just because it existed millennia before even the first traces of what is called 'history.' That, however, is a subject that we need not offend with in this book, beyond saying that it was a period before this descent of *manas*, a period, that is, before the human ego with its separative and consequently strife-engendering vision had become manifest, and which, therefore, offers no parallel to present conditions.

As things stand now there can be no interaction between the spiritual perception of the *buddhi* and the physical perceptions of the senses, except through the instrument of *manas*, the focal point between the two, the two-faced Janus who looks before and after, above and below, and is consequently a mirror which can reflect both Hemispheres.

The Self may thus be compared to an astronomer who seeks to make a chart of the stars that he sees above him in the heavens. In this analogy, the unchanging heavens above correspond to the ideal pattern of the Upper Hemisphere as depicted in the *buddhi*, the telescope to *manas* and the chart to the world of sense. Having focussed his telescope he gazes at the heavens and then endeavours to depict their pattern on his chart. Having succeeded in setting down a few of the stars he saw, he again looks back to the heavens and then once more returns to his chart.

In just the same way there is or should be a rhythmic in-looking and out-looking in our lives. As psychologists would express it, after a period of introversion in which we view the inner archetypes of being, there comes a corresponding period of extroversion during which we try to see those archetypes as manifest in the outer world. The one should succeed the other with the same regular rhythm as that in which out-breath follows in-breath. This is a fact we too often forget, and, favouring one or other of the modes according to personal temperament, we endeavour to concern ourselves with only one of the two worlds, either that of 'matter' alone, or, though less frequently, that of 'spirit' alone. The interplay of both is necessary if we are to have psychic health. We may call the two modes, theory and practice, or vision and action. Vision must come first if right activity is to follow but a vision that is not translated into practice goes negative and sterile, like breath that is retained too long in the lungs.

But we are leaving out the question of the instrument, the *manas*, which has an independent life of its own, one which causes our astronomers a great deal of trouble. In the first place, dust and moisture collect on the lenses and have to be carefully wiped off. "For mind is like a mirror; it gathers dust while it reflects. It needs the gentle breezes of Soul-Wisdom to brush away the dust of our illusions." In the second place, having, as we have said, a life of its own, instead of 'stay-

ing put' in the same focus while the astronomer re-
produces the pattern on his chart, it wanders off in search
of aims of its own, and so, when the next period of
in-looking comes, much of the allotted time has to be
spent in re-focussing before any further progress can
be made.

The duty of *manas*, then, as an instrument, is to re-
sign its own life into the hands of its user: "Lord, into
thy hands I commend my spirit." It should be a
window through which the lower can perceive the
Higher and the Higher manifest itself in the Lower.
Hence the stress that has been laid in all Yoga on the pu-
rification, the stilling and the concentration of *manas*.

For *manas* is indeed the inner Door which leads to
the Higher Worlds. It is true that there are other
ways of gaining knowledge of those Worlds; drugs,
for instance, and the hypnotic trance of mediumship.
Those ways, however, are not a going through the Door
but a violent breaking through the walls and it was to
them that Christ referred when he said:

"He that entereth not by the door into the sheep-
fold, but climbeth up some other way is a thief and a
robber. But he that entereth in by the Door is the Shepherd of the sheep......Verily I say unto you, I am the
shepherd of the sheep. All that ever came before me
are thieves and robbers; but the sheep did not hear them.
I am the Door: by me if any man enter in, he shall be
saved and shall go in and out and find pasture. The
thief cometh not but to steal and to kill and to destroy;
I am come that they might have life and that they might
have it more abundantly."[1]

This passage, as should be entirely clear, has a
profound inner meaning: the psychikoi, those who are
called *bālāḥ* or 'children' in this Upanishad, into

---

[1] *St. John's Gospel*, Chapter 10.

whose hands it fell, have characteristically made of it a sectarian attack on all other Teachers than their own.

Christ, as all should know, is the Godhead's voluntary 'descent' and 'sacrifice', the putting on of human limitations in order to be the Door or intermediary between the Lower and the Upper Worlds.[1] Hence his crucifixion on the Cosmic Cross, for the central point of the two intersecting lines is just *manas*. It was not as a personal Teacher that he contrasted himself with 'those who came before' but as symbolising the unique Door of the higher *manas*, the Door which furnishes the only safe method of going in and out if life is to be healthy and 'abundant.' All other modes of communication between the inner and the outer are harmful to the Soul and in the end produce nothing but loss and destruction. It was as that Door that Christ proclaimed that he must be "about his Father's business" and said "not my will but Thine be done."

We must return, however, to our text. A question is often asked as to who is the actual experiencer of life, or as the Upanishad calls him, the *Bhoktā* or enjoyer, he who is bound by good and evil deeds. The horses of the senses are, though living, unintelligent, and the *Ātman* is universally admitted to be forever free and blissful. Who or what is it, then, that becomes entangled in the experiences of life? The answer is that it is neither the *Ātman* nor yet the senses but that *Ātman's* Light as reflected in *manas* and sense. Just as the reflection of the sun in a mirror takes on an individuality of its own and is distorted by the irregularities of the mirror, so the Light of the *Ātman* is reflected in the mirror of the *manas* and becomes a self or separate being. If that mirror is controlled by the harmonious order of the *buddhi* all is well, but, unfortu-

[1] Compare the *adhiyajña* of Gita 8. 4.

nately, it is usually not the "gentle breezes of Soul-Wisdom" to which it opens itself but rather the fierce and distorting gusts of sense desire. Hence the image is a distorted one, and, since the harmonious alone can be free, it is by that very distortion bound and entangled in the reactions to which it gives rise.

All Light and all Life is the Light and Life of the *Atman*. There is no other. But, if the *manas* reflects that Light on the world of sense alone and not on the heavens of *buddhi*, the resulting life is that which we call a personal or lower self, an experiencer of actions who is inevitably entangled in their results. Hence the teaching in verse that the *Ātmik* Light together with *manas* and the senses, but without the ordering pattern of the *buddhi* is that self which is the experiencer of life here below, the self which is in bondage and is in need of 'liberation.'

That self is in truth only a partial manifestation of the one harmonious Self, and, being partial, it is said to be 'unreal.' Nevertheless, though unreal, it can be intensely painful. Its incompleteness renders it certain that while it persists, it shall be, as the Buddha taught, 'a Burden Bearer,' the Golden Ass of Apuleius, for whom life is indeed but endless sorrow.

How then can freedom come and who is freed? The *Atman* is for ever free, and we, the lower selves, for ever bound. Where are the magic Rose-leaves by eating which we may regain our true Human shape and freedom? Once more we are brought back to *manas* which is the very crux of life.

"We" are essentially the point-like spots of the Creative Light reflected in the *manas* and in us is the Divine Freedom to look up or down. If, lured by the glamour of sense, we look down and forget the upper and divine half of our being, the starry harmony of the *buddhi*, that harmony retires into the darkness and "we," the conscious selves, are left with only half of our true being and that the lower half. We have become lower selves wantoning like runaway children in that outer sunlight which is darkness to the true Seer. If, on the other hand, we look upwards to the Stars—and the result of ignoring their guiding light is to experience such grievous disasters that, in the end, life itself forces us to do so—we can once more regain the unity, of our divided being, and, ceasing to be 'lower' or 'burden-bearing' selves, become once more those Higher Selves which, behind all the false appearances, we have never ceased to be.

There is in truth but one Self and that unmanifest; its manifestations may, however, either be partial, one-sided and so 'lower' selves, or unified, harmonious higher Selves. There are no entities called lower selves which can evolve into the Higher. As the Buddha taught, the personal self is something quite 'unreal' and can never 'evolve' into anything else, or attain *Nirvāṇa*. There are, however, distorted manifestations and there is harmonious manifestation. On the ceasing of the one, the other is revealed. We may remember the Gita's twin definition; Yoga is skill in action: Yoga is harmonious balance (*samatva*).

That *manas* may be said to be enthroned in Yoga which exerts no self-will of 'its own' but is a perfect focus or balancing point between the Upper and the Lower Hemispheres, through which, as through a true lens, the Light of the Higher can shine forth into the Lower. Thus the latter can regain its lost Divine Harmony and the Golden Age shine forth once more, this time with the added beauty of self-consciousness. Assuredly Yoga is by no means the selfish 'soul-saving' affair that it has, by some, falsely been supposed to be.

Not individual 'salvation' but 'God's Kingdom' is the aim of all true Yoga. The mind in Yoga is a diamond point in which are alike reflected the Heavens above and the Earth beneath.[1] From their marriage arises the new Heaven and Earth, "for the former heaven and earth have passed away" and the reflecting mirror of the mind, expanding to the frontiers of infinity, becomes itself the All that gave it birth.

The text, therefore, describes two types of man. The first is one who is without the synthetic, unifying vision of the *buddhi*, without it, that is, in the sense that he has turned his back on it and gazes only downwards at the alluring images of the sense world, to the reflection of which his mind gives itself over utterly. Such a man is, as we have seen, only half a man. Lacking one half of his being he is unable to stand upright but leans over perpetually in response to the pull of the senses; hence he is continually forced to be on the run if he is to avoid collapsing. This being constantly 'on the run' is what we call the force of desire which thus brings it about that he is for ever seeking outside himself for the lost half of his being, that which, in reality, he has left 'behind' or 'within' himself. Conscious of his lack of completeness, he perpetually seeks for it where it is not, in the glitter of gold, in the idle voice of fame, the intoxication of personal power or the seductive arms of lust. Always the sought-for goal beckons mirage-like from the far horizon, and always it vanishes as the disappointed traveller reaches the spot where it seemed to be.

Nor is that all; nor is it enough that he should wearily climb the treadmill steps of mere outwardness. Under these circumstances, as the Gita tells us, Self is the enemy of self. That higher Half of his being that he has turned from pursues him with all the fury of a woman

---

[1] Compare the Buddhist *Vajrabimbopamā Samādhi*, the Poise like the Diamond Point. See *Abhidharmakosha*.

scorned. As Artemis the Divine Huntress, the cold Moon of Fate pursues him with relentless arrows which pierce his undefended back with their keen points, and, ever and again, sounds forth the baying of her hounds, hungry as they follow on his trail. He is on the point of success and is stricken down by illness; power comes within his grasp but something intervenes, perhaps a scandal of his long-past youth which comes to light 'by chance,' destroying men's confidence and so his chance of power over them. Even in the arms of what he knows as love he is not safe, for always something comes to thwart the happiness that seemed about to come. "All things betray thee who betrayest Me." And all the time the baying of the death-hounds grows louder while slower and slower fall his tired feet. Gradually his strength fails as the life-blood ebbs away from the wounds in his back made by the deadly arrows. No longer are heard the trumpet notes of his triumphant outrush, those bugle notes that set "wild echoes flying." Now only echo answers "Dying, dying, dying!" His vision begins to fail. No longer can he see the lights of sense that drew him, those fire-flies of the marsh that aped the eternal stars, so that, in the end, he sinks exhausted on the ground and the hounds of the remorseless Fate which is himself come up speedily, and, destroying with their gaping mouths his personal form, bring about an enforced return to that unity of being which he has so long denied.

But not in this negative and enforced manner can the true unity be attained. For the time being an end has no doubt been set to his striving but he has left outside him that which will not for long allow him to rest. The outer world is still full of the ghosts of his desires, ghosts which can neither rest themselves nor let him rest. Each object of his past desires became filled with the life which he projected on it, and now,

like ghosts, they wander round his head calling for
him to take again that life. The sorcerer who evokes
spirits and forces them to serve him, becomes himself,
at death, their slave and hard is the service they exact.
Now no longer they but he is the one to be evoked:
they call and he must follow.

Hence is it that the spirits of desire that he has
left behind him now call him forth once more with
power that was his own. The magic words are spoken,
and, though he sleeps, yet sleeping, he must once again
go forth to do the bidding of his past desires. Thus
he must once more leave the inner Peace and, with a
grim inverted resurrection, pass through the Gates men
call the gates of birth but which the wise know are the
entrance to the Tomb.[1]

Thus he who has ignored the voice of the *buddhi*,
turning his back upon its message of unity, and whose
mind is in consequence impure with the uncontrolled
forces of desire, "does not reach the Goal but wanders
in the Ocean of the World," the Ocean of repeated births
and death, drinking the bitter water of its waves that
only serves to increase his thirst yet more.

Opposed to this picture is that of the other type of
man, he whose *manas* is harmoniously poised (*yukta*)
between the Upper and the Lower Hemispheres. In
the mental mirror of such a one the outer world of sense
is seen as the reflection of the eternal stars above. Within him and without, all is one. When he looks within
he sees, not darkness, but the Guiding Light of that
Divine Harmony, and, when he looks without, he sees
that same pattern reflected in the still waters beneath
his feet. Hence for him there is no unbalance in the
mind, no leaning over and no frenzied running. All
is for him one harmony of which he forms a part. The

[1] The Orphic initiates termed the physical body the Tomb.

horses of his Chariot indeed may move with the independent life with which in the past he himself endowed
them. Nevertheless the reins of a harmonious *manas*
are fastened to their mouth and the other end of those
reins is in the firm hands of *buddhi*. Move they must
and will, but only in the direction that is desired by
the calm far-seeing eyes of the Divine Charioteer. No
lures of wayside grass and fleeing mares can take them
from the Path chosen by the Driver, nor free them
from the iron grip with which he holds their heads.

Such is the type of chariot that reaches the End
of the Road, one of which the Horses are controlled
by the reins of a purified *manas* held in the Divine hands
of *Buddhi*. In plain language, he who would reach the
Goal must see that his senses are controlled by his
manas or self-conscious mind. He must at all times
practise what the Buddhists term *samyak smriti*, right
recollectedness, or attentiveness to what is happening.
He must keep a careful watch on the workings of his
senses, analysing their complex patterns into movements that are useful and movements that are useless
or even harmful: the former he must encourage and
the latter discourage. It is just this task for which
manas is fitted, its central position as the self-conscious ego ensuring that all the different strands of
sensation come to one focal point where its bright and
analytic vision is able to disentangle and examine
them, especially with reference to the causes from which
they arise and the effects to which they give birth.

But this task it can by no means accomplish if
it attempts to stand by itself in independence of that
which is higher, for, in that case, its judgment will be
swayed and moulded by the lower forces of sense, to
which, as we have seen, if it forgets the Upper Hemisphere it inevitably leans over. Only ho who has carefully watched his mind and its workings has any idea

of the extent to which his apparently free and self-originated decisions are but the dancing of a marionette pulled from beneath by the invisible strings of desire. That is the Fate to which we expose ourselves when we ignore the Divine Levels of our being.

Therefore, if the *manas* is to perform its proper task of controlling the senses, it must itself reflect the ideal pattern that is laid up in the heavens of the *buddhi*. Only when that pattern is reflected in its mirror from above has it a standard of reference by which to judge the separate acts and sensations that are reflected from beneath. It is this that the Teacher means by being united with the *buddhi* and by having the intuitive judgment or *Vijñāna*.

Nor should we think that the possession of such a divine standard by which to judge is an attainment that is far above us; one to which perhaps we may aspire in some dim future. Here and now the Pattern is within us, within all of us, within everything that exists, man, animal, plant or stone.

It is in fact immanent in every atom of the universe had we but eyes to see it. Nor is it in truth the eyes that are wanting. Having eyes we see not. For ever it shines before us; it is the habit of attending to it that we lack. We have *forgotten* it, and the forgetting, like all such, has been deliberate, a forgetting that is motived by desire, the desire to be independent and to go our own way free of all control. It may be categorically affirmed, indeed, that all disbelief in the Higher, in the Divine, in what is usually called 'God,' however plausible may be the reasonings which seem to support it, arises in just this way, in order that we may feel free to go our own way, to follow blindly our own desires. 'God' stands for ever before us. We do not see him because we shut our eyes, preferring the so-called freedom, which is really enslavement to the senses, to the real freedom which is service of the one Divine Harmony. We will not see 'God' in front of us and therefore are compelled to feel a 'Devil' behind. This is seen everywhere today for *manas* is the keynote of the present age with its so-called modern civilisation. Everywhere man seeks freedom from the restraints of a past that he does not see is really his own self. Everywhere he demands freedom to choose for himself which means to make a choice that is unrestrained by the Spirit but which is none the less fettered by Desire, the sinister relentless Fate that is the manifestation of that Spirit when ignored. There is no freedom in Desire, none, none, none. Men desire wealth and Fate brings them poverty; health and it brings them sickness; unity and it brings them separation; peace, the selfish peace of getting their own untrammelled way, and the Spirit brings 'not peace but a sword,' the sword which is now, at this very minute, at the throats of the nations.

Only in a life that is lived in union with the Spirit can there be freedom, happiness or peace. Never, as long we, individually or nationally, seek to ignore that Spirit and its divine harmony, shall we attain that serene poise of soul in which is alone true freedom and true peace.

It is useless to say that we do not perceive that divine pattern. We do not because we *will not* see it. Just as, when seeking to point out a faint star, the teacher directs our attention first to a bright one that is near it, so when seeking to point out the subtle harmony of the *buddhi*, he first directs our attention to the voice of conscience which, as we have already seen, is its manifestation on a lower scale, a manifestation that is *to us* brighter because existing in what is Day to us though Night to him. Whatever anthropologists or Freudians may say, the voice of conscience *is* the

Voice of 'God,' or at least its reflection, dimmed for
our purblind eyes. By submitting the patterns of sensation to its ordering control we rise from the lower
to that higher *manas*, which, poised on the frontiers
of Day and Night, can hear the Soundless Voice itself
and see the Divine harmony of the Starry Gods reflected in its calm and limpid depths, just as, even in broad
daylight, the stars can be seen in the depths of a really
deep well. By the steps of conscience let us descend
that well, the central well of the Heart to which we have
already referred more than once. In it for ever shines
the Pattern with whose aid we can even now attain the
Knowledge, which being known, requires no other:
the key to that serene and God-like life of Freedom,
that Divine Memory which Plato writes of and which
Arjuna triumphantly proclaims[1] at the conclusion of
the Gita, the Philosopher's Stone, the Universal Medicine, that One Thing, in fact, which, under one name
or another, has been the object of all sacred quests
throughout the ages, the One Thing which is the
"Strength of all Strengths," and "the cause of per-
fection throughout the whole world."[2]

This One Thing is called by the Teacher the
Paramapada or Highest State of Vishnu, that Living
Spirit which pervades the whole, and which, as the
Vedik mantra tells us, is seen by the wise pervading
all things like the Light of Day. This designation
is particularly to the point since it is by uniting
with the unifying, all-embracing vision of the *buddhi*
that it is attained. When by its aid the Cosmos is
no longer seen as a chaos of separate selves and separate things but as one all-enfolding harmony in which

[1] Gita 18. 73. "Destroyed is my delusion; Memory is attained."
[2] The Emerald Tablet of Hermes.

each is all and all is each, where "each contains all within
itself, and at the same time sees all in every other," where
"the Sun is all the stars, and every star again is all the
the stars and Sun,"[1] then, indeed, has the chariot arrived at the End of the Journey: all that remains is
the final Flight, alone on the Swan's Path through the
Upper Air, a Flight in which the now useless chariot is
left behind and the naked Spirit soars beyond Sun, Moon,
and Stars to the Unmanifest Beyond.

(10)   *Higher than the senses are the (subtle) objects of*
                                                            sense;
       Higher than those objects is the mind (manas);
       Higher than manas *is the* buddhi;
       Higher than buddhi *is the Great Self*
                                              (Mahān-Ātmā).

(11)   *Higher than the* Mahat *is the Unmanifest;*
       Higher than the Unmanifest is the Purusha,
       Than the Purusha *there is nothing higher.*
       That is the End,[2] *that the ultimate Goal.*

In these verses the Teacher goes on to describe
the hierarchy of principles, the Ladder of Being that
reaches from Earth to Heaven, the Ladder up which,
like the angels in Jacob's Dream, the Souls descend and
ascend.

The lowest rung of that Ladder is formed by the
senses (*indriyas*) which represent the ordinary level of
normal waking consciousness, and, on the objective
side, the ordinary world of sense objects that we see
about us.   Higher than that, we are told, is the level

[1] Plotinus 5. 8.
[2] Literally the Pillar, which marks the farthest end or boun-
dary. Beyond it is only the No-thing, the Great Void.

of the *arthāḥ* usually, translated as the objects of sense. The question at once occurs, however, why the objects of sense should be considered higher than the senses which perceive them. Surely the two are on the same level, or if there is to be any preference, it should be given to the senses rather than to their objects. The fact is that, as Shankara points out, the *arthāḥ* are not here the objects of sense, trees, stones and what not, that we see but the subtle forms which may be called their psychic archetypes and which bring it about that the objects of ordinary sense perception are what they are. There could be no seeing of red, for instance, in the outer world if there were not a subtle redness within the psyche. We can perceive nothing 'outside' ourselves that we do not first possess 'inside' and the world without is but the manifestation of the subtler world within. As Hermes says "it is true, certain and without falsehood that what is below is like to what is above"; like to it because it is its reflection or manifestation. However strange it may seem to some, it is a plain fact which he who cares to can experience for himself that this oppressive outer world, this "too, too solid earth" is a phantasmagoria, a projection of the subtler inner world as truly and certainly as the picture on the screen is a projection of the slide in the magic lantern. The earth we tread on is not solid and resistant because of any quality itself possesses nor does water flow because of any 'fluidity' of its own. It is, as we have said, true, certain and without falsehood that the earth is solid because it manifests the element of solidity that is in the psyche, and water is fluid, or the sky blue for precisely the same reason. If it were not for this inner world of archetypal sense elements there would and could be no world of outer perception at all.

Moreover, it is the existence of this inner subtle order that is, at least immediately, responsible for that regular order of nature that scientists make so much fuss about, for the fact that, relatively speaking, we all perceive much the same world outside us. It is true that this only takes us one step back but it is at least a step in the right direction, and, if followed up as in our two verses, will lead to the ultimate source of the cosmic order in the *Rita* or Divine Harmony. Ultimately the Cosmic Order is an imagined and willed order, an order that exists in Consciousness. It is, on a given level, more or less common to all men simply because 'all men' are moments of that Consciousness, and, though each sees the Order from his own particular point of view, each such vista or perspective (to use Russell's term) is necessarily interlinked with every other. Proximately, as we have said, the outer order takes its rise from and reflects the subtler one that our text refers to as that of the *arthāḥ*, or subtle elements of sense. Incidentally these inner sense elements are not matters of mere philosophical conjecture. They can be perceived directly by the inner senses that all have but which few either understand or pay attention to. They are, in fact, shining in what Paracelsus refers to as "the Light of Nature which is shining before the eyes of every man, but which is seen by few mortals."

Nor are we referring particularly to the visions of a few exceptionally constituted people that we call clairvoyant. The inner senses of all men are acting here and now—if they were not, we should not perceive this world at all. As in the case of the *buddhi*, so-called civilised men have more or less deliberately forgotten to attend to them. Among what are called primitive and uncivilised men even today, their use is common and well known. Nothing in fact interposes so great a barrier between 'primitive' men and the anthropologists who seek to 'understand' them as the fact that the former make use of two sets of senses and the latter only of one. All very ridiculous no doubt, but a fact nevertheless.

"I am the Master of Balliol College
What I don't know isn't knowledge !"

The sooner, in fact, that European 'civilised' man gives up this conceit the better will be his understanding of other peoples and the sooner will he regain his inner health.

In any case, it is for the above reasons that the *arthāḥ* are said to be 'higher' than the outer senses and their world. They constitute what has sometimes been termed the astral plane, in Hindu tradition the state of *swapna*, the intermediate or *Bhuvar Loka*, which we shall here refer to as the World of Desire. It must be remembered that what we are dealing with are levels of experience and what we have seen so far is that higher than that level which we call the ordinary physical world is a subtle inner world, the world of the inner sense objects, the world of Desire.

Higher than that again is the level of *mānasik* experience, corresponding to *manas* in ourselves. On that level the content of experience, the so-called sense data, outer or inner, are all referred to the central point of self and so form patterns around that point. Being thus related to 'me' they become 'mine' and form the content of myself. It is on this account that the objects around us, instead of flowing freely through our being like water through a sponge, get held up and fixed, thus becoming 'property.' This process is essentially the same whether the objects in question are tables, chairs, houses and what not, or whether they are what we term our physical bodies. The former class of objects in fact become an extension of our physical bodies and the attachment to them is very often no less than that to the latter. The loss of our property is an affliction that is different only in degree from the loss of our bodies, and, in earlier times, crimes against property were treated as almost identical with crimes against the person.[1]

All this is due to the centralising and integrating action of *manas*. Nevertheless, we have so far looked at this principle from its unsatisfactory and negative, but unfortunately too common, side. Its activities have, however, another aspect as well, for *manas* is essentially twofold.

"The *manas* is said to be twofold, impure by contact with desire and pure when free from it. *Manas* is indeed the cause of both bondage and liberation for men; of bondage when attached to objects, of freedom when unattached."[2]

These two aspects are, of course, our lower and higher *manas*, the two modes of the one integrating principle. The real trouble with the 'lower' mind is not that it produces an integration, a self, but that it is an unbalanced, incomplete and so a false self. Forgetting, as we have seen, the higher half of being, it leans over in one direction and from the wealth of the entire universe selects only a limited portion for its integration. This, of course, produces a self which is not the true centre of being, but which is removed from that centre to a greater or less extent and which we may represent as in the diagram below:

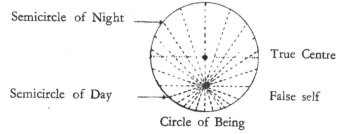

Semicircle of Night

True Centre

Semicircle of Day

False self

Circle of Being

[1] It is not much more than a century since in England a man might be hanged for the theft of a sheep.

[2] *Maitri Upanishad* 6. 34.

The result of this unbalanced integration is of course that a stress is set up and is always pulling on the self and being resisted by it. This pull is what is known as the pull of Fate, the resistance, the 'instinct' of self-assertion and self-preservation, the urge to preserve the integration at all costs. Hence the false ego attempts to rush outwards, away from the true centre of its being which becomes an object of fear to it, something that menaces its very existence, something whose pull must be counter-acted in every possible way. This is the reason for that fear of the inner life which is so often found among us, the reason why ordinary worldly men, those, that is, who are clinging with all their being to the outer circumference, are apt to apply the term morbid to all inward-turning. They are right; morbid means that which leads towards death and for them the pull to the centre is the pull of death. As long as the self succeeds in maintaining its resistance to the central pull, so long it continues to live its separate life. Sooner or later, however, its forces begin to wane, and, losing its grip on the outer edge of being, it sinks back to the centre and dies.[1]

We have already seen, however, that the path of Yoga is a voluntary death. We can now understand why that must be so and why Christ said "Ye must be born again." As long as the distorted and partial self remains, so long there can be no freedom from the pull of Fate and no inner happiness. The grip on the external must be voluntarily released and the self be dissolved into the dark centre of being before the true and balanced integration of the New Birth can take place.

[1] It is not intended to imply that after death it remains in the centre. It certainly passes *through* that centre, hence the traditional and real importance of the death moment, but pendulum-like, it swings over to the other side, the dark half of the circle of Being. The above account is highly simplified.

Thus self must die before Self can be born.

This New Birth is the birth into the higher *manas*, the true centre of our being. It was symbolised in Egypt by the birth of Horus and in India by that of Kartikeya, the Eternal Youth, the son of Fire, who, nursed by the Pleiades, the microcosmic Seven, rides on the Peacock of the Starry Heavens, his twelve hands showing forth his mastery of the twelve-fold Wheel of Fate. In Taoism, it was the blossoming of the Golden Flower and it is referred to in *Light on the Path* as the Flower that blooms in the silence that follows the storm.

Flowering as it does at the true Centre of being, there are no distorting forces working upon it. Harmoniously its lotus petals extend to the furthest edge of the waters of life, open alike to the Sun of Day and to the Moon of Night. Serene it stands, floating upon the Waters, not held in place by any force or violence, for, being in the true centre, there is nothing to disturb its poise, and it is therefore "firm as the (also unsupported) earth is firm, calm as a mountain lake."[1] No more has it any attachment to 'property,' for property involved the existence of what is not 'mine,' and now all things within the Universe are calmly held within the shining mirror of its heart. It has indeed attained all possessions, but those possessions are such as "belong to the pure soul only and are possessed therefore by all pure souls equally." Hence is it that it has also "the sacred peace which nothing can disturb, in which the soul grows as does the holy flower upon the still lagoons."[2]

Such is the higher *manas*, the soul of the disciple who has passed through Death to Life and now will die no more.

But this voluntary Death and re-birth cannot be attained without the aid of something higher than mere

[1] *Dhammapada.*
[2] *Light on the Path.*

manas. Left to itself, the *manas* knows no order, no harmony, but its own partial and distorted one. Outside that order everything is the blackness of chaos and therefore, as we have seen, it clings to its own integration, which, however partial and therefore full of suffering, is yet preferable to being swallowed up in the belly of the monster which its own one-sidedness has brought to birth in the dark Waters. Hence there are real dangers on the Path, for, if it loses its present integration without being able to attain the new, its disintegration will be that catastrophic swallowing up that we term madness. From this fate it can only be preserved by the Guru, the Divine Harmony of the *Buddhi*, which alone can watch over the soul's helpless state while self is being transformed into Self.

This is why faith (*shraddhā*) in the Guru, inner or outer, or rather both, is so essential, for true faith is, as we have seen, reflected knowledge of the Cosmic Order. Such a faith can serve as the Guide, for its reflection of the Divine Harmony hovers over the Waters and thus can lead forth the New Birth from the dark chaos into which the old self has been melted or dissolved by the operation of the Secret Fire. Hence the care with which the secret of that Fire has always been guarded and the universal injunction that it should never be revealed except to a fit disciple, for if one without Faith in the Guru should attempt the dissolution it could only end in terrible disaster. The sinister powers that his previous one-sidedness had called into being would utterly devour the rash adventurer and, instead of the Divine birth of Kartikeya under the "sweet influences of Pleiades," there would result a brood of monstrous births under the opposite sign of the Scorpion, a demonic brood, hungrily warring amongst themselves for the possessions of the scattered limbs of what was once the self. Such a state is what men know as madness, the most deadly of all the perils on the Path. "Whosoever doth approach unpurified," says Agrippa, "calls down judgment on himself and is given over to the devouring of the evil spirit."[1] Therefore a second warning is written over the Gateway: "Only he who has true Faith in the Guru should set foot within." In the Guru alone can be found salvation at this juncture and therefore the text states "higher than the *manas* is the *buddhi.*"

Faith, we saw was the reflection of the Divine Harmony, *Buddhi* is the clear-eyed perception. Higher therefore than the perception of the Harmony is the Harmony itself and therefore we read: higher than the Buddhi is the *Mahān Ātmā* or Great Self. This Great Self or *Mahat* is itself the Cosmic Order, the great Brahma-World, the Soul of the manifested universe.

In later writings, such as those of the classical and scholastic Sānkhya, *Buddhi* and *Mahat* were fused together and counted as one principle. Our Upanishad, however, preserves the earlier tradition in which *Mahat* is the substantive Cosmic Order and *Buddhi* the perception of that order by *Manas*.

Buddhi is indeed the Moon of Wisdom, the Mother Isis, who, wedded to divine Osiris, gives birth to Horus, the Son. In the Hindu symbolism she is Saraswati, Goddess of Harmony, whose husband is Brahmā himself. She is the Eternal Virgin from whose womb is born the Son of God, Devaki, "in whom are all the Gods,"[2] giving birth to the Divine Krishna in the dark prison created by Kansa, the lower self. She is equally Mary, the Virgin Queen of Heaven, bringing forth Christ in the dark stables of animality. The *Buddhi* has thus a twofold role, symbolised and manifested in

[1] Agrippa: *Three Books on Occult Philosophy.*
[2] *Srimat Bhagawata.*

the two eternal roles of woman, motherhood and wife-
hood. Seen from below, she is the Mother of the new-
born God, but from above she is the Bride of the
Father, and dwells for ever in sacred union with Him
in that Brahma-World or plane of *Mahat* of which she
is indeed the 'lower' half. It was therefore not without reason that the mediaeval Catholic Church taught
that the Virgin was the intercessor between man and
God nor that it clothed Her in the Blue star-spangled
Robe that Egypt knew of as the Veil of Isis. In all lands
and in all ages the one eternal Wisdom is the same.

In any case we can see why it was that in some
systems the *Buddhi*, as the Bride of the Father, was
reckoned as one principle (*tattva*) with Him and included in the name of the Great Principle (*Mahat tattva*)
or the Great Self (*Mahat Ātman*) while in others, and
especially in such as are concerned with the Divine Birth,
she as the Mother of the Son, was reckoned separately
—"Higher than the Buddhi is the Great Self."

The "Great Self" is the wide-extended Brahma-
world, the Cosmic Egg which includes within its shell
the totality of manifested being. It is in the most
fundamental sense the Cosmos, for all lower worlds
are partial views, abstractions as it were, from that all-
inclusive Whole. From one point of view it is the
Father of all, or even, as Hindu tradition puts it, the
Grandfather (*pitāmaha*), reckoning ourselves as the Sons
of our Higher Egos and those Egos as sons of the
Great *Brahmā*. But in itself it is the Son of the Nameless Being beyond, the Divine Son who springs from the
union of *Purusha* and *Prakriti*, the unmanifest Sun and
Moon, the two Poles into which the Ultimate One
divides and which are, as the Gītā tells us, eternal
moments of its being.[1]

[1] *Gītā* 13. 19.

Chapter III

Our Upanishad is not directly concerned to give an account of the great cosmic origination, so we shall confine ourselves here to as brief a statement as will suffice to explain our text.

The Root of all is the dark unspeakable Being (or non-beingl) of the *Parabrahman* to which words can not reach. From the testimony of Seers, however, we know that even in the Night of *pralaya* "that One Thing breathless, breathed by its own nature."[1] This Breath, the ultimate life-breath of all Worlds, brings it about that the two eternal Poles into which its unity divides, the *Purusha* or Pole of Subjectivity, and the *Prakriti* or Pole of Objectivity, now, with the 'Out-breath,' become overt, and now, with the 'In-breath,' remain latent.

These two Poles form a duality, the ultimate Duality of the universe; but, as the severed aspects of one Whole, they unite once more in outwardness and the fruit of that Sacred Marriage is the Son or *Mahat* which partakes of the being of both. From its Mother, the *Prakriti*, it derives its unthinkably rich content, that content which has caused it to be described as the Treasure House of the Universe, and from its Father the Spirit or *Purusha*, it derives the Golden Light with which it shines and to which it owes its name of *Hiranyagarbha*, the Golden Germ. Moreover, as a unitary being, it is the bright and outer reflection of the ultimate dark Unity of the *Parabrahman*, of which, indeed, it gives us whatever knowledge we possess, since, as Christ said, "He who has seen the Son has seen the Father" and he who has seen the Shining Golden Germ has, in a sense, seen that which can never be seen, the Black Fire of the ultimate Brahman which burns for ever beyond the frontiers of the Cosmos.[2]

[1] Rig Veda X. 129. 2.

[2] This statement of Christ's has more than one level of mean-

With the birth of the Golden Germ, the manifest universe comes into being. We may even say that its being is, in a sense, complete at that stage since it contains all that is or ever will be manifest and all 'lower' worlds and subsequent experiences are rather differentiations or stratifications of its infinite riches than any new manifestation or 'Creation.' As for its Golden Light, that shines alike on all that takes form within the Egg whether that form be of a God, a man, an ant, a plant or even a stone.

After this brief excursion into cosmology we can return to our text which tells us that "higher than the Great One" is the *Avyakta* or Unmanifest, a term which, though belonging in a sense to all that is beyond the *Mahat*, is more particularly applied to the universal Matrix known as *Prakṛiti* or *Mūla-prakṛiti*, the great unmanifest Mother, from out of which, by the shining of the Light, all form and all content whatsoever emerges into manifestation. Just as the *Buddhi* is the manifested Mother who gives birth to the Higher Self so is the *Prakṛiti* the unmanifest Mother from whose dark and fertile womb emerges the Cosmic Son.

As within the dark bosom of the earth in winter lie buried countless seeds which spring to life as all the rich variety of plants that come forth under the rays of the northward moving Sun, so within that dark womb lie *in potentio* the seeds of all the countless beings that will under the Sun of *Puruṣha* emerge into differentiation in the warm sunlight of the Cosmic Day. Therefore it is said that beyond the Son is the Mother, the Great Sea that even yet nurses in its dark depths, "stranger

ing. The personal self is the 'Son' of the Higher Self and that Self the 'Son' of the Great Self or *Mahat*. Thus Christ's words indicate to us a ladder leading from our ordinary waking selves to Ultimate *Parabrahman* itself. Truly, as the Oracle of Apollo proclaimed, "Know Thyself" is the gateway of all wisdom.

fish than ever came out of it," the source of nourishment for all the universe, the Horn of Plenty, pouring forth its gifts in a ceaseless stream.

Some schools of thought, claiming the authority of Shankara, have depreciated the Great Mother and called her 'only *Māyā* or *Avidyā*,' ignorance. *Māyā* indeed she is, for where is Māyā like a mother's, and the term *Avidyā* as applied to her means primarily the dark abyss of *non-being*[1], and, secondarily the mysterious darkness of the unmanifest state, a darkness that, we should not forget, may mean Night to the ordinary man, but is Day to the Seer. It may also be remembered that it was not till Shankara had composed a magnificent hymn, the famous *Waves of Bliss*, to the Universal Mother, that he was made free of the Path that lies beyond.

That Path beyond is the *Purusha*, He who dwells in the *pura* or City of the Mother. As She is the Moon of Night and secret Wisdom, so He is the Sun of Day and open knowledge. When 'together' in the Cosmic Night She is the New Moon who eclipses the Sun, while, when 'separate' during the Day, She is the Full Moon shining in opposition, her whole being illuminated by His rays; though sometimes, indeed, the shadow of her child the Earth intervenes, and, eclipsing the Sun, causes a false night to descend upon us.[2]

He is the Light of Knowledge, She the dark depths of Wisdom: He the Fountain of Unity, She the dark wealth and richness of plurality, the fecund ocean that is

---

[1] *Vid* means both to be and to know.

[2] Notwithstanding the finger of fun which is so often pointed at the 'oriental astronomer,' sitting with the pen of his accurate mathematical calculations in one hand and the conch of his 'superstition' in the other, there is a deep significance in eclipses which is quite unsuspected by the modern mind. Moreover, they *are* connected with a Dragon, though we shall pursue the subject no further here.

the mysterious womb of life.

From one point of view these two great Principles, both of them in themselves unmanifest, are on the same level in the hierarchy of being, and, like Sun and Moon, weave out the rhythmic pattern of their mystic interaction on the path of the same Ecliptic. From another point of view, however, the Sun or *Purusha* is considered 'higher,' both as the Source of the Light that we value, and because His unity appears nearer to the Ultimate One than does the diversity or duality. This, however, may be to some extent an illusion, apparent only from our point of view which sees unity as more ultimate than plurality. In itself the Ultimate *Parabrahman* is not one but rather O, the mystic zero, the Great Void of the Buddhist Schools. Such a zero is in truth equally and indeed infinitely distant from all the numbers. It is no 'nearer' 1 than 2 and we may also note that the term *advaita*, usually loosely rendered as monism, means actually non-dualism which is not quite the same thing.

All the same, from our point of view, a certain priority has to be conceded to the Unity of the Father-Light or *Purusha* for it is that Light that, reflected down here as it is on all the levels of the Universe, constitutes the Path by which we reach the goal. It is over that Rainbow Bridge of Light that our steps must take us. It is the Light which, reflected in all beings high or low, we must trace from the gross to the less gross reflections, from the less gross to the subtle and from the subtle to the deep divine. For what we seek is *conscious* liberation. To have reached the dark Mother is indeed to have reached ultimate being and there have been those who have attained that blissful state known in Hindu philosophy as *prakriti-laya* or absorption in *prakriti*, the state which is reflected in the bliss and freedom of dreamless sleep. Nevertheless, if it is a conscious and illuminated freedom that we seek, and indeed such an attainment is as near as we can go towards describing the meaning of the whole cosmic process, we cannot rest content in the bosom of the Mother but must continue following the thread of Light that has been our guide through the labyrinth of being and trace it back, even 'beyond' Her, to the Sun who is its Source. That Sun is the *Purusha*, higher than which as the Teacher tells us is nothing at all, words that once more have a hidden sense.

As far as anything can be *named* as the Goal, the ultimate *attainment*, it is the *Purusha*, referred to in verse 13 as the *Shānta* or Peaceful *Ātman*, the calm and tranquil Eye of the Universe, which, like the sun, gazes alike on the just and on the unjust, on the good and on the evil sides of universal life. To have reached it is to have finished the course, to rest serenely on the Farther Shore of being, in the Fearless, Sorrowless state. It is the summit of the Mountain, or rather, for the Golden Germ is that, it is the Light of Heaven that broods in utter peace above that Summit. Beyond It there is nothing, nothing, nothing; and should one seek to circumnavigate its infinite sphere he would return at once to his own starting point. Therefore it has been called the final goal, the Ultimate Limit.

And yet the words which say that there is naught beyond bear, as we have said, a hidden meaning. True there is nothing beyond, no-thing beyond and not even a 'beyond' in which to seek. Nevertheless there is the mystic Zero, Shunya or Nothing, within which the Light of Unity and the Darkness of Duality alike abide, the Dark Fire in which are both Light and Darkness, the utterly unspeakable That, the O from whose mysterious 'centre' wells up during the Cosmic Day the whole series of numbers, the 2 no less than the 1.

Of that Dark Zero, nothing can be said, nor indeed can any reach it during the Cosmic Day. Those who have reached the Goal have gone to the Father-Sun of the *Shānta Ātman*. Beyond it none have gone and none shall go till the coming of the Night. It is the Goal, we need talk of no other. Beyond it there is nothing, nothing that we, or even a God, can name. As Lao-Ise has it, "The Tao which can be named is not the true Tao."

(12) *Hidden in all beings this* Ātman *is yet not visible. It is to be seen, however, by the keen and subtle* Buddhi *of those who are Seers of the Subtle.*

The *Purusha* of the last verse, the transcendent *Ātman*, though (as being 'beyond' even the unmanifest *Prakṛiti*) it is not in itself manifest, is yet concealed in the very heart of all beings down to the very atoms and electrons. It is the concealed Life of all that is, both of what we term living beings and of what our academic ignorance terms inorganic or dead matter. In itself, like the light which is its symbol, it is invisible. Only when it illuminates and is reflected in some form does it become visible in the same way as a beam of light in a dark room becomes visible only if there are particles of dust or other matter in the air. Note that objects of sensible magnitude, though themselves lit up, do not suffice to show the beam which illumines them. That can only be done by the relatively subtle dust or smoke, the particles of which are sufficient to make manifest the beam without at the same time obstructing its passage. In the same way the gross objects of this physical plane, even the most minute, are themselves illuminated by the *Ātmik* Light which has called them forth from their unmanifest condition in the Darkness, but are too obstructing or *tāmasik* to reveal the passage of the Light Ray. That Ray can only be seen in the subtle and purely *sāttvik* objects of the *Mahat*,

which, reflecting but not obstructing, its passage reveal
it to those who are able to make use of the keen far-
seeing and subtle vision of the *Buddhi*, those who
have raised their consciousness to the higher rungs
of the Ladder of Being that was described in the two previous verses.

(13) *The Wise should dissolve Speech in the* Manas
and that (manas) *in the Knowledge-Self* (jñāna ātman, i.e.,
buddhi). *That Knowledge-Self he should dissolve in the
Great Self* (Mahat) *and that in the* Shānta Ātman *or Peaceful Self.*

Having understood the nature of the Ladder and
its various rungs "the Path whose foot is in the mire,
its summits lost in glorious light Nirvanic,"[1] the
disciple must now tread them one by one. The Ladder
commences of course in the senses, in the 'mire' of
which its foot is planted. The word Speech in the
verse is, as Shankara points out, "used illustratively
to denote all the senses" of which as a correlation of
sound and so of *Ākāsha*, it is the highest and subtlest.
We have already said that the Light of the *Atman*
is present in everything, even in the world of sense,
and, indeed, it is by that Light that the sense objects
are seen. Therefore, the first step for the wise disciple
is to learn to discriminate the unchanging Light from
the changing objects of sense that it illumines. This is
the process of *Atmānātmā Viveka* or discrimination between Self and not-self as taught by the Vedānta; it is
also the alchemical process of distillation or sublimation by which the subtle portion of the matter in the
retort is driven off by heat and so obtained in a purer
state. Instead of forgetting or taking the Light for

[1] *Voice of the Silence.*

granted and becoming absorbed as do most men in
the sense objects which it illuminates, the disciple must
learn to pay attention to the Light itself even though
at present he will only be able to 'feel' and not to see
it. Attending to it in all his every-day perceptions,
he must gradually identify himself with it rather than,
as heretofore, with the physical body which was for
him the most important of the sense objects. In reality
that body is but one of the many objects illuminated,
but, since it is always present in our experience while
other forms come and go in endless succession, it has
come to be that part of the sense world with which
we particularly identify ourselves.

That identification must be broken. First from the
outer objects and then from 'his own' body he must
dissociate the Light, and, ceasing to consider himself
the former, he must identify himself with the latter.
This is called dissolving the senses in the *manas* for, as
we have seen, *manas* is the seat of personal and individual self-hood. Whatever *manas* identifies itself with
is felt as self. Actually the process has two stages, that
of the gross physical senses and their objects and that of
the inner or subtle senses of verse 10. The work having
been successfully achieved with regard to the gross
sensations coming from the world of outer objects,
it has to be repeated with the subtle and desire-toned
images of phantasy that make up the world of the inner
or 'astral' senses. From them too the Light must be
withdrawn so that neither they nor their outer counterparts have any longer the power (given to them originally by us ourselves) to make us feel enriched in being
with their coming or impoverished at their going away.
"Nothing of mine is burning there," said King Janaka
as he watched the flames eat up his capital.

Even with a little practice of this discipline the disciple will become aware of a difference in his con-

sciousness. As Sri Krishna said, "Even a little of this Yoga delivers from great fear."[1] The forms of the sense world, both outer and inner, will of course remain with him, but there will be a change in his attitude towards them. No longer will they smash their way brutally into his being. They will be found to have lost their sting, their power to wound and enslave the consciousness, which will, indeed, watch them come and go with the detached interest with which a man watches a crowd pass by his window, their shapes and characteristics no doubt noted with interest but neither their coming longed for nor their departure feared.

Gazing on the world in this way, a calm will descend upon his spirit, the calm which comes from severing "with the axe of detachment" the ropes of self-identity that bound him to the forms. No longer feeling his heart-strings tugged at by all that come and go, he will be able to repose serenely in himself and this is called dissolving the senses in the mind. It is also termed separating the mind from the body. If it is asked how it is that these two apparently quite different statements mean the same, it is replied that it is that portion of the self that is identified with and lost in the sense objects, that is withdrawn or separated from them and which is to be united with or dissolved in the *manas*.

At the same time, he will find that his power of dealing with the outer world has increased and not decreased. By no means need he or should he become a mere introverted dreamer of dreams, helpless before the problems of practical life. "Yoga is skill in action" and his practical skill should increase and not decrease as the result of being able to see things as they really are instead of, as always before, through the distort-

---

[1] Gita 2. 40.

ing glasses of desire and aversion.

The Buddha rightly termed this part *ehi-passika*, a 'come and see' Path, and the Gita the Path of direct Knowledge.[1] Even from the very commencement, he who treads it correctly will experience in and for himself the reality of its fruits so that gradually he will be liberated more and more from the necessity of relying on the external 'authority' of books and teachers. His own Teacher is a different matter, for the latter is not without but within himself and will be with him till the End.

Having withdrawn his self-projections from the objects of sense and reunited them in the mental centre of his being, he must now repeat the process and climb higher. He must ask himself who is this self, this mind, this I, which seems to be so separate from all else. Following up the same clue he will observe, first in the calm periods of meditation and then habitually, even in the midst of action, that what he calls his self is actually a certain particular pattern of sense and mind data, certain thoughts and habits of thought, backed and enriched by sensation and desire, but all lit up by the one Light which he has now learnt to recognise. His self in fact is a seeing and thinking of the world from a particular angle or point of view and it may again be divided into a seen World and the Light by which the seeing is done. Again he must distil off or separate out that Light which he will find to be a Light that is not in any sense 'his' but one which is universal in all men, the Light of 'others' no less than of 'himself.'

This time, however, the process of distillation is a harder and more subtle one. 'He' has to pass beyond 'himself' and how should he do so? To what should his hands cling while raising his lower limbs from the

[1] Gita 9. 2. *pratyaksha avagama.*

170

mire in which they were sunk? Up till now the task has been relatively easy. Enthroned in the very castle of 'self' hood he has only had to strengthen that self by cutting it loose from all that weakened and entangled it. He has had the lure of enhanced self-mastery to spur him to the effort. How shall he proceed further?

Nowadays, especially in the West, there are many who are interested in and even practise Yoga up to this point and for this very attainment. The bait which has drawn them is that of enhanced self-hood and well-being, of increased self-mastery with its corollary of increased mastery of the outer world. So they come to this point and then stop; for why should they go further? Beyond this point is the other-worldliness of the ancient East, a thing for which the average modern man has little if any use. He may indeed consent to sit at the feet of Eastern teachers so far as gaining increased self-hood and enhanced life-efficiency is concerned but beyond that he will not go. Indeed he makes a virtue of this half-heartedness and proclaims aloud his conviction that the Western way of life, rooted in selfhood, has in it something far superior to any dreamy eastern trans-individualism. Again and again this attitude can be seen in Western writers otherwise sympathetic to Yoga; in the writings of psychologists such as Jung and of those who follow so-called purely western and occultist traditions. Jung for instance says that we should do well to confess that we do not understand the utter unworldliness of a text like this; indeed, that *we do not want to understand it.*[1]

There are also some western occultists who would agree with Maitland's remark that the Western system "represents ranges of perception......which the Eastern

[1] Introduction to Wilhelm's translation of *The Secret of the Golden Flower.* Italics mine.

has yet to attain." Another well-known western occult writer urges that the ego must undoubtedly be preserved for practical reasons and will have nothing to do with any dissolution that might 'take place at the expense of the ego.'

These statements illustrate the difficulty which we have referred to, that of passing beyond the dead-centre of the ego. So long as a yogik technique or discipline can be used for the strengthening and aggrandisement of the ego, for just so long will the modern man (who lives for and from his ego) practise it if once convinced of its usefulness for that purpose. But to follow it up beyond the ego—that is another matter altogether: the whole Pandora box of modern inventions is invoked as a witness that that would be too much of a good thing.

Nevertheless to stop at this point is really to fail in the Yoga and to reduce the latter to the status of one of the many modern devices for increasing the comfort of man's ego; to place it, in fact, on the level of an airliner, a wireless set, a new vaccine or a psycho-analytic panacea.

To all such we would say "if you don't want the goods don't muck 'em about." Stick to your beloved ego and leave us our Yoga in peace, for Yoga is a sacred science which leads far beyond the realm of modern conveniences and psychological adjustments. He who wishes to stop short at the stage of a glorified ego has entirely failed to understand the real nature of the Path which is one that must be trodden, not for any benefit that may accrue, but for its own sake and for love of the Eternal if we are to avoid a terrible Nemesis that lies in wait for him who prostitutes the sacred Science for worldly and ego-centric aims. This path is the Path of Death.

Beyond the separateness of *manas* is the unity of

buddhi and therefore through the *manas* to the *buddhi* we must follow the Light. "I would," says Hermes to his disciple, "that thou hadst even passed right through thyself," a thing which is impossible as long as it is for the self that we are acting. Our Upanishad gives us no information as to how this passage through is to be accomplished, but, supplementing its teaching with that of the Gita, we can say that the one force capable of taking man through the bottle-neck of self into the wide-extended regions beyond is the force of love or *bhakti*, the one force in the universe which is capable of driving out all thought of self. It is on the wings of self-giving that the further reaches of the Path must be followed up.

The preliminary step is of course the discrimination of the thoughts and ways of thinking which make up the pattern of the mental self from that which is the thinker of those thoughts, the Light which holds them in being and on whose waves they float. The discovery is then made, as we have already said, that that Light is a universal Light, one which is equal and the same in all beings, something that is no more 'me' than it is 'you'. From the point of view of that Light the self to which we have so fondly clung is but an inter-linkedness of thought-data, the famous 'knot of the heart'[1] which has to be unloosed, a dead thing which, for all the extravagant value we have set upon it, is really an obstruction in the path of free Light flow.

The Light is the only Life and if we are to speak of Self at all (the Buddhist tradition refuses to do so) it is in that Light that true Self-hood lies, a Self-hood that is not separate in you, me and him but one in all. It is to that Light that we must transfer our real being, thus separating spirit or *buddhi* from *manas*, or, in the other

---

[1] *Muṇḍaka Upanishad.* 2. 2. 8.

way of speech, separating out the Light of Self that was entangled in the knot of *manas* and uniting it with or dissolving it in, the all-pervading Light of the *Buddhi*.

The means by which this task is to be accomplished have already been indicated. The Cosmic and divine pattern of the *buddhi* must be taken as the guide for all actions, feelings and thoughts. Not for the sake of self but for the sake of the Whole must all be done and felt and thought. The Inner voice that now sounds loud and clear must be accepted as the Guide in everything so that the pattern of life may become a harmonious reflection of the divine Harmony instead of, as heretofore, a selection from that whole for the purposes of the separate self. This task, however, can only be accomplished if we call to our aid the great power of Love, in some form or other, usually that of utter devotion to the Guru. Naturally the self resists its disintegration and only by the help of and for the sake of 'another,' as the Teacher has already told us, can the work be successfully carried through to the next stage. "The same am I in all beings" says Sri Krishna, speaking as the one Guru, the *Buddhi*, and adds "They who serve me with devotion, I manifest Myself in them and they unite their being with Me."[1]

In him who utterly makes over the pattern of his life into the hands of that Divine Guru, the latter manifests himself. Slowly but surely the old one-sided pattern is destroyed and the new and all-embracing Pattern takes its place. In the now calm waters of the *Mānas* lake the Eternal Stars shine in living splendour. Under the influence of those rays the transmutation takes place and it was for this reason that Paracelsus taught that he who would achieve the Elixir of Life must

---

[1] *Gita* 9. 29.

know the *sacred* science of the Stars; for it is by their Light that the transmutation is accomplished and the crystal waters of the Elixir collect like dew in the empty vessel of the heart.

Thus is achieved the dissolution of the *manas*, or self of opinion, into the *Buddhi* or Self of Knowledge.

Concerning the next two stages we shall say little, for he who has travelled thus far has surer guidance within himself than any written words could furnish. We will merely add a few lines for the sake of that intellectual completeness so beloved of the mind.

The penultimate stage, the dissolution of the *buddhi* in the Great Self of *Mahat* is scarcely separate from what has gone before. The Stars that shone reflected in the *Mānas* Lake have accomplished their purpose of translating that Lake to their own Heaven so that its waters have become the Living Heavenly Waters that well up from within the Foot-print of *Vishṇu*. As an ancient inscription said to have been found in Egypt has it:

Heaven above, Heaven beneath;
Stars above, Stars beneath;
All that is above is also beneath;
Understand this and be happy.[1]

The *Buddhi*, the Heavenly Bride, adorned in the jewels she has salved from the bitter ocean depths, hastens of her own accord to rejoin her Lord, the *Atman*. Their Sacred Union makes up the wondrous being of the Great Self.

"Those to whom all this experience is strange may understand by way of our earthly longings and the joy we have in winning to what we most desire—remember-

---

[1] Quoted by Eugenius Philalethes in *Magia Adamica*.

ing always that here what we love is perishable, hurt-
ful,......There only is our veritable love and there we
may hold it and be with it, possess it in its verity, no
longer submerged in alien flesh. Any that have seen
know what I have in mind......Thus we have all the
vision that may be of Him and of ourselves, but it is
of a Self wrought to splendour, brimmed with the
Spiritual Light, become that very Light, pure, buoyant,
unburdened, raised to Godhood."[1]

Beyond is the tremendous brooding calm of the
transcendent *Shānta Ātman*, of which, as Plotinus tells
us, if we think of it as Mind or God, "we think too
meanly." To it there are two ways. The first is that
on which all knowing and knowable are deliberately left
aside: "every object of thought, even the highest we
must pass by......in sum, we must withdraw from all
the extern, pointed wholly inwards; no leaning to the
outer; the total of things ignored, first in their relation
to us, and later in the very idea."[2]

The total of things is of course the great Whole
of the Brahma-world, the true or Divine Universe.
Even that Divine and wondrous Being must on this
Path be renounced and left behind or dissolved, the
naked Spirit soaring ineffably, "alone to the Alone." For
him whose Spirit travels by that road there is no return
whatever, nor any possibility of extending aid to those
whose souls still welter in the bitter waves below.
The Bright Fire is extinguished in the Black Fire of the
Unmanifest. The Light has mingled with that Light,
which, though in itself the Light of Lights, to us is
Darkness.

"He is become a portion of that loveliness which
once he made more lovely," and, though in some mys-

---

[1] Plotinus 6. 9.
[2] Plotinus 6. 9.

terious sense, the entire ocean is slightly sweetened by
his Flight yet there remains no possibility of aid from
him for us as individuals here below. It is the
End.

On the other road there is no willing of the final
Flight. Out of the Marriage of the Sun of the Great
Self with the Moon of *Buddhi* is born by the upward
birth a Divine Son who has his being in the *Shānta
Atman* beyond, a Son who is greater than his Parents,
but who, born of love, does not abandon them, but
rather watches over them from Beyond. Or, to put it
in another way, the Bird of the living Spirit is set free
by the love-embrace of the Sacred Pair and Soars above
them into the Empyrean. Thence as a Divine Genius it
watches unseen over the destiny of the Pair beneath,
whose Essential Heart is thus enthroned in the utter
Freedom of Transcendence while still an outer being
is maintained to carry out the Divine Work here below.
This is the Secret Path, the Path of Love.

We can say no more. All that we have said is but a
bridge of words which will crumble into dust at a touch.
It will just serve, however, for him whose feet wear
the winged sandals of Hermes and who is fearless enough
to leap and look not behind. Then, if it crumbles into
dust *behind* him, what matter? Its purpose has been
served.

(14) *Arise! Awake! Having attained to the Great
Ones understand (The Path). Sharp as a razor's edge is
that Path hard to cross and difficult to tread: so say the Seers.*

The teaching about the Path having thus been set
forth, the Teacher urges his pupil to arise and "strike
his tent," to awake from the night of ignorance that
rules in the lower planes of the cosmos, and, in Plato's
phrase, to "flee to the beloved Fatherland."

12

He has attained to the direct view of those Great Ones, the Teachers who are yet one Teacher, and whom he has now met "face to face" and "light to light." He is now one who is "able to stand, able to hear, able to see, able to speak, who has conquered desire and attained to self-knowledge, who has seen his soul in its bloom and recognised it and heard the Voice of the Silence."[1]

Confidently the Soul stands upon its own feet with eyes that are open to behold the Divine Stars, ears that can hear the soundless Harmony of the Spheres. In these days when those who sit in the shade of the Tree of Knowledge can scarcely be discerned in the glare of the outer sunlight, any one who has reached to this point and attained knowledge of the Path that has just been described is apt to be made a Mahātmā of, or even deified by those who are fortunate enough to come into his orbit. Fortunate is it for him if he is not himself deceived by the acclamations which ring in his ears. In earlier ages his position would have been more accurately judged. He has in fact trodden one half of the Path, for to have met the Teacher face to face is not the same as to become himself a Teacher, and to have heard the teaching of the further reaches of the Path is not the same as to have trodden them. Half the Work has been accomplished; half remains yet to do.

Therefore the Teacher urges him not to be satisfied with what has been achieved, nor turning round, to be content to shine, a brazen sun amidst a circle of leaden planets, but to make the most of the opportunities he has now gained, to penetrate into the very heart of the Teaching he has received. He is to *understand* with the magical 'understanding' of the heart the Path that stretches before him, and, having understood, to tread it firmly to

[1] *Light on the Path.*

the end.

It is a difficult Path indeed, sharp as the edge of a razor, the almost inconceivably subtle Middle Way that leads between the two Poles to the very Heart of Being.

The slightest loss of balance at the dizzy height at which he now stands will have disastrous consequences undreamt of at lower levels. Moreover, at those heights, there is a great Wind that blows perpetually, and, though unlike the gusts below, its pressure is a steady one, yet it is only too easy for the disciple to lose his head and be whirled away from the knife-edge ridge he treads, back to depths from which he will have painfully to climb again.

The tension is terrific and constant. One outburst of anger that would scarcely be noticed in the dense air below will give rise in that rarefied atmosphere to an explosion which will shake the very depths of his being and undo in a few moments the painful efforts of months or even years. One longing gaze towards the safety of the valleys he has left will provoke a dizziness of the head which may send him headlong to rejoin them. "Kill in thyself all memory of past experiences. Look not behind or thou art lost."[1]

The ordinary rules of ethics, those mass-produced books of words that are adequate enough as guides in the populous valleys, are quite useless or even misleading at these lonely heights. Within himself the disciple must find the harmony which alone can guide him and any mistake will be a cash transaction, a thing for which he must pay then and there. Let him meditate on the fact that if he has six virtues he must have six vices

[1] *Voice of the Silence.*

to balance them;[1] and if this hard saying arouses fear or confusion in his mind, let him not venture far from the crowd or he will surely perish.

Things are visible at these heights that are mercifully invisible below. The Spirits of the Air, "the jealous lhamayin in endless space," are no longer a dim tradition or an old wives' tale but an ever-present reality, and, though they can do no harm to him who fears them not, they can cause the timid soul to lose irreparably its precarious balance.

"Beware lest in the care of Self, thy Soul should lose her foothold on the soil of Deva-knowledge."

"Beware lest in forgetting SELF, thy soul lose over the trembling mind control, and forfeit thus the due fruition of its conquests."

"Beware of change! For change is thy great foe. This change will fight thee off, and throw thee back, out of the Path thou treadest deep into viscous swamps of doubt."

......"Prepare and be forewarned in time. (But also) Remember, thou that fightest for man's liberation, each failure is success, and each sincere attempt wins its reward in time."[2]

Assuredly, as the Seers have taught, it is a difficult and dangerous Path, one which many have sought and failed to find, many have found and failed to tread and some have trodden successfully to its glorious end. At least we may remember the words of Sri Krishna:

"Neither in this world nor in any other is there destruction for him (who treads this Path)."[3]

(15) *Having realized that* (Ātman) *which is soundless,*

---

[1] Said by H. P. B. to one of her pupils.
[2] *The Seven Portals.*
[3] *Gītā*, 6, 40.

touchless, formless, tasteless, and without smell, permanent,
without beginning or end, greater than the Great One (Mahat),
Fixed, one is liberated from the mouth of Death.

In this verse which carries on the thought of the
last we are shown why it is that this Path is such a difficult one. The *Shānta Ātman* is utterly transcendent,
entirely free from those sense qualities by the help of
which we recognise and identify objects. How, indeed,
are we to know 'that which is devoid of all the distinguishing marks by which we know things? We can
only do it by the path of negation, by rejecting in all
experience all the qualities which sense perceives, and,
it may be added, all the characteristics which the mind
thinks. What remains when this has been done is the
Light which supports them all equally, the Light of the
Ātman. The sky is full of clouds but it is not to any
cloud that we must give our attention. Rather, we
must strive to realise what it is in which the clouds are
floating. But in truth, as Plotinus said, our way takes
us beyond knowing. The *Ātman* is not an object of
any sort that can be 'known' by a subject. It is itself
the eternal Subject and consequently anything to which
we can point, anything which can be known as such,
is not that *Ātman* but, at best, its reflection in something
else. The *Akāsha* in which the clouds float can only be
'known' when we can *feel* the clouds floating in our
own being, when, that is, we have ourselves *become*
the *Akāsha.* When we can feel ourselves that mysterious and apparently characterless being in which
forever float all the images of sensations and thought
that make up the universe, then and only then have
we identified our being with that of the *Ātman* and then
only can we be said to 'know' it. No other type of
knowledge is possible. As another Upanishad puts it
"how should one know the Knower," save, of course,

by being oneself that Knower. Nor, having 'known' it, is any verbal description possible to which objections cannot be taken. Such words as are used in the text are but an attempt to express the nature of the experience and must be taken as such.

It should not be forgotten that the *Atman* is not something which is far away, "pinnacled high in the intense inane."

It does not "lie away somewhere leaving the rest void; to those of power to reach, it is present; to the inapt, absent. In our daily affairs we cannot hold an object in mind if we have given ourselves elsewhere, occupied in some other matter; that very thing must be before us to be truly observed. So here also, preoccupied by the impress of something else, we are withheld under that pressure from becoming aware of the Unity; a mind gripped and fastened by some definite thing cannot take the print of the very contrary."[1]

The 'something else' that prevents our seeing the *Atman* is of course the *content* of experience, the vivid images of sense and even of thought. These are what we attend to and to which we give ourselves. Hence we fail to feel the *Atman* in ourselves, or, to speak more correctly, we forget to identify our being with it.

For the *Atman* is here and now in all experience, even the most trivial. Its full realisation may be a "far-off divine event" for us who think in terms of time, but it is present *now*; without it we could neither write nor read nor understand these words or any others. At the very back of our being, now at this moment, its Light is shining and by that Light we see and taste and touch and feel and think. It is of the very utmost importance that *now* we should turn back to what we have forgotten, for in that alone is our true being, a being

[1] Plotinus, 6, 9, 7.

that is beyond this and all other universes (greater than the *Mahat*) and which, when discerned, is known with an utter certainty, surpassing all we count as knowledge, to be imperishable, without beginning or end, the one Fixed thing in all creation's flux.

> "It ascends from earth to heaven, and descends again, new-born to the earth, taking unto itself the power of the Above and the Below. Thus the splendour of the Whole world will be thine and all darkness shall flee from thee.
> This is the strongest of all Powers, the Force of all forces, for it overcometh all subtle things and can penetrate all that is solid. For thus was the world created."[1]

And again: "The First Principle doth consist in an unity and through rather than from this is all power of natural wonders carried into effect......Those who are ignorant of this Principle......had they mastered all the books of the wise, were they conversant with the Courses of the stars, did they clearly understand their virtues, powers, operations, and properties, their types, rings, sigils and their most secret things whatever, no working of wonders could possibly follow their operations without a knowledge of this Principle."[2]

He who has known it has found the Universal Elixir: he is delivered from the Mouth of Death.

(16) *By hearing and repeating this ancient tale of the Nachiketas Fire,[3] taught by Death himself, the wise one*

[1] *The Emerald Tablet* of Hermes.
[2] Trithemius of Spanheim, quoted by Vaughan in *Anima Magica Abscondita*.
[3] Usually translated as 'this Nachiketas story,' but it is the account of the Nachiketas Fire and not of Nachiketas himself that

becomes great in the Great World of Brahma.

*(17) He who repeats in purity of heart this supreme se-
cret in the great Assembly (or the assembly of the wise)
or at the time of offerings to the dead is destined for the Eternal.*

These two verses conclude the first half of the
Upanishad and indeed may even at one time have con-
cluded the Upanishad itself. At any rate the three
chapters which follow are somewhat in the nature of a
supplement.

It was customary to conclude treatises with a verse
or two expressive of the value of the teaching contained
therein and often, also, enjoining secrecy upon the reci-
pient. It is not to be supposed, though, that he who
could write this Upanishad would be content with the
conventionalities of mere formal praise.

The 'hearing' and 'repetition' which referred to and
which are signs that the hearer is on the Path are not of
course the formal repetitions of orthodox ceremonial.
The 'hearing' is the hearing from a competent Teacher
which takes place when the pupil is ready and the
repetition is the manifestation in the pupil's own life
of the truth he has heard. The Great Assembly of the
Wise is the fellowship or brotherhood of those who have
gone before upon this Path and into whose ranks the
disciple now enters as a neophyte. All other links are
now severed and in the depths of his soul it is to that
brotherhood alone, the deathless "Race that is never
taught," as Hermes terms it, that he is now united.
Hence the prophecy as to his future destiny.[1]

was "related by Death." Similarly the *Brahma sansadi* of the next
verse is usually translated "an assembly of Brāhmaṇas." *True* Brāhmaṇas perhaps; but as *brahma* also means great, we have preferred
the above rendering. Compare also the *Turba Philosophorum.*

[1] Compare the Buddhist tradition about the prophecy made

Chapter III

The reference to funeral ceremonies is not hard to understand when we remember that the teaching is concerned with the Path through the gates of Death. The *Shrāddha* ceremonies were not always the mere formalities that they usually are nowadays. Those who had knowledge were able to assist the departed soul on its journey through the inner worlds and in such a connection this text, when transmitted from the mind of the 'living' reader to that of the still present though invisible 'dead,' would, like the ancient Egyptian Book of the Dead and the Bardo Thodol still used in Tibet, serve to guide the soul on its wanderings and enable it to make the utmost use of the strange circumstances in which it found itself after the loss of its body.

by Dīpankara Buddha to him who, ages after, was to become Gautama Buddha. See *Introduction to the Jātakas*.

CHAPTER IV

We now commence the second part of the Upanishad which, as we have suggested, is possibly an addition or supplement to the first part. Not, however, that it is any less true or authoritative in the only real sense of that much abused term, for its authority is precisely the same as that of the first part, the authority of truth, experienced and realised by the unknown writer. Just as the first three chapters gave us the teaching about the Path, its difficulties, and the method of treading it, so these last three impart to us the Knowledge, as far as it can be imparted at all, which arises in the heart of him who treads it faithfully. It is only to such a one that this knowledge is or can be of any real use. Mere intellectual philosophers may, if they please, dissect it and make it the subject of their learned discussions but they will gain nothing from it except its husks; for the words, even the most abstract and philosophical of them, are symbols and refer to experiences quite beyond the range of academic philosophers. Such experiences are only known to and therefore only comprehensible to him who is treading and has in part trodden the Path already described.

(1) *The Self-evolved One* (swayambhū) *pierced the sense-openings outwards; therefore one sees what is without not what is within oneself. (Occasionally) some wise man, seeking Deathlessness, with reversed gaze has seen the Inner Self.*

(2) *The* *childish follow after external objects of desire and therefore they enter the wide-extended snare of*

death. But the wise, having known the Deathless State, seek not the Fixed Pole of being amid the transient things of this world.

The Self-evolved one, the Great Being known as *Brahmā*, whose dwelling is the universal Lotus that has sprung from the navel of the dark and unmanifested *Nārāyaṇa*, is said to have pierced the openings of the senses outwards. This is not an operation performed on the unfortunate souls on some Brāhmik operating table but just a statement of the fact that all cosmic manifestation is a gazing outwards, away from the true centre of being. *Brahmā* as the One Life of all gazes outwards and does so from each point of his being. Each such point thus becomes an individual self, an individual centre in the one being, which, gazing outward, sees all its fellow selves as outside and separate from itself. "As above, so below." This out-turned gaze is manifested on the physical plane in the fact that all the normal sense organs are as it were holes pierced in the skin of our unity and so give us information of what is outside that unity. Only the inner sense sometimes known as intuition, the faculty that gives us knowledge of the unity, does not thus manifest through an outer aperture but remains "concealed within the hollow of the brain," its very existence unknown to the out-gazing crowd of men.

The sense organs are of course not the senses themselves, for the latter are living spiritual Powers, Gods in fact; but there is a correlation between them, and the external apertures in the skin are the expressions of the outgoing nature of those Gods, the real senses.[1]

The result of this outward-turnedness or extraver-

---

[1] The more ascetic schools might perhaps demur and say that

sion is that we perceive only that which is outside an
separate from ourselves, a world of separate selves an
objects, in the midst of which, incomprehensibly enough
we find ourselves placed. Our backs are turned toward
the wealth of bliss, the riches of the Divine univers
within, and we vainly seek outside for a happiness tha
exists only within, the dim memory or feeling of whic
is what gives the edge to our seeking.

What we can see with our physical eyes is real: wha
we can grasp with physical hands is alone a positiv
attainment. Such is our attitude toward life and to th
touchstone of these physical senses we bring everythin
that we may know whether it is real or 'merely ima
ginary.' It is difficult for us to realise that all that w
see in the outer world is but a projection of the divine
ly imagined universe within, but so it is in truth. Eve
the very word *kalpa* used for a Day of Brahmā, signi
fying as it does something that is imagined, shoul
teach us where it is that we must look for the true realit
of what appears without.

In the Chinese book of yoga already referred to i
is said "If for a day you do not practise meditation, thi
Light streams out, who knows whither? (and then
the primordial spirit is scattered and wasted. Whe
it is worn out the body dies......The meaning of th
Elixir of Life depends entirely on the backward-flowin
method."

Similarly, our text tells us that occasionally som
wise man or other, in search of that Deathless State tha
all men who have not entirely sold their birthright for
mess of pottage know to exist somewhere or othe
dammed up the outflowing Light of consciousnes
and turned it back towards its source within. This

the senses are Devils rather than Gods but *demon est deus inversus* at
Gods are by no means always benevolent to fools.

the backward-flowing method that the Chinese teacher
refers to, and, as he says, "it has nothing to do with
an actual looking within." In other words, it is a withdrawal or reversal of the flow of *Consciousness* and not
any squinting of the eyes as practised by some *haṭha
yogis*. Our consciousness normally flows outwards
through the senses to the objects which it illumines
and then proceeds to lose itself in those objects.
Thus it forgets even its own existence and we have the
extraordinary sight of learned thinkers actually denying
that any such thing as consciousness exists at all.

    This outflow must be checked if Deathlessness is
to be achieved and the stream of Light be directed back-
wards into what seems at first the dark inner abyss from
which it takes its rise.

    As long as we allow our Light to flow out into ob-
jects of desire and bind ourselves to them by the bonds
of attraction and repulsion, so long that Light is identified with the objects and seems to share in their
transiency. When in time the objects change and
pass, when they are destroyed as all objects must be
sooner or later, the Light which is bound up by identification with them seems to vanish too, and, as the
text says, we walk into the wide-spread net of Death.

    The wise, however, knowing of the Deathless Being
within, no longer seek for the fixed Pole of their being
amidst the outer flux where nothing at all is or can be
fixed, but, withdrawing the self-projections that have
bound them to the objects, enter, as has been said, the
dark interior cave of being. Within, at first, is nothing
but darkness and there are many who, after one hasty
glance, conclude that all is emptiness and gloom
and hurry outwards again into the delusive sunshine
of life.

    If, however, the disciple persists in his endeavours,
if, rejecting the outer brightness, he makes the dark his

constant dwelling place, his in-turned eyes will get accustomed to the blackness and in the midst of it, a far-of
point of Light, the Pole-star of his being, will begin to
shine and light the Path for him. That Star which is
the star of his Inner Self, will grow brighter as he advances towards it and by its beams he will be able to distinguish the true from the false. As long as he remains
beneath the sphere of the Moon, so long the drifting mists
raised by that luminary will cause the light to twinkle
uncertainly, but once he has passed beyond, it will become steady and grow in size and brilliance until it has
become the very Sun of his being, the deathless Light
that is his true Self.

This Light has indeed always been present. It was
this and no other that lit up the outer world, for, as the
next verse tells us.

(3) *That by which one knows form, taste, smell, sound
and mutual contacts, what remains here (when all these
sensations have been eliminated), this verily is That (Ātman
that transcendent deathless being about which thou hast en-
quired).*

(4) *Having recognised that Great and pervading Ātman
by which one sees both in waking and in dream the wise one
grieves no more.*

Were it not for this inner Sun there could be no
light in the world at all. After it and not before it comes
all the business about electro-magnetic waves and what-
not, after it and not before it the lenses, optic nerves
and brain structures. By that Light one sees, hears and
touches, by that Light one thinks, by its rays, even, one
questions its own existence. "The fool saith in his
heart there is no God" and yet it is by the power of
God that the thought is framed.

By that Light we perceive the world of waking

experience and by that same Light all the objects of
our dreams. All that we see, waking or dreaming, are
but images floating in that sea of Light, images that have
no substantiality at all. Nowhere is there any true solidity in the worlds of sense, outer or inner. Thinner
than the surface of the thinnest soap bubble is the world
which confronts us. Its apparent solidity is but borrow-
ed from the soul; it is the firmness with which we have
anchored our souls in the forms. Draw in those an-
chors, sever those chains of attachment and the solid
earth vanishes beneath our feet, the eternal rocks dissolve before our eyes and walls of stone and steel no more
obstruct our passage than the filmiest wreaths of mist.
For the Great Ones no obstructions can exist. Christ
appeared suddenly in the midst of closed doors. Apol-
lonius of Tyana removed his limbs from chains to show
his doubting disciple that it was but his own will that
kept him in Domitian's prison, and similar events have
been recorded even in recent times.[1] Those who have
gone far enough on the Inner Path know with a certainty beyond all cavil that this "too too solid earth" can
and does "thaw and resolve itself into a dew" and that
nothing in it can obstruct even for an instant the passage of the free soul.

Therefore it is that none who has seen clearly that
Light of the Great Pervading Soul can ever grieve or
feel himself imprisoned in a hostile world of matter.
He has seen with calm immortal eyes the walls of matter
pass like summer clouds and he knows with an utter
certainty that nothing can ever bind him except with a
power that he himself bestows upon it. This is no
mere metaphor or poetry, no merely 'spiritual' or
after-death promise, but a plain fact and to this day there

[1] For example Trailanga Swami of Benares within living
memory.

are those living in our midst who know and will bear witness to the fact that what has been written above is the plain truth.

(5) He who knows this Honey-eater, the Ātman, as the (one) Life, ever near, the Lord of past and future, thereafter, he shrinks away no more. This verily is That.

The *Ātman* is here referred to as the Honey-eater, a word which is usually taken to mean simply the enjoyer of pleasures, the sweets of action. It does no doubt mean that but much else besides as those will know who are aware of its use as a ritual drink in many of the ancient mysteries. The honey-clover was connected with Osiris in Egypt and the *Brihadāranyaka Upanishad*[1] gives an account of the *Madhuvidyā* or Honey wisdom which was obtained with great difficulty by the *Ashwins*, and of which the final teaching was:
"This *Ātman* is honey for all beings and all beings are honey for this *Ātman*. This shining deathless *Purusha* who is in this *Ātman*, who is indeed this *Ātman*, he is just this *Ātman*: this is the Deathless, the *Brahman*, the All."
We may remember, too, how, in the Gita[2], the *Jīva* or Higher Self is described as leaving the body at death and taking with it the subtle essences of the senses as the wind takes scents from flowers. This also is one reason why bees and butterflies have often been used as symbols of the Soul and sheds light on the famous riddle of Samson "out of the strong came forth sweetness."
The *Ātman* is in fact the ultimate Subject of all experience, and, whereas the personal self 'feeds' on the

[1] 2. 5.
[2] 15. 8.

gross sensations, it is only their Honey or subtle essence that is assimilated by the *Ātman*. Therefore one must seek within oneself for that deeper being in the six-sided cells of which the Honey of all experience is stored. Within our personal selves, those ephemeral creatures of a summer day, is stored the Honey of countless ages, stored up to be the food of the dark winter months of withdrawal. But who or what is it that integrates that store into a whole, that makes a unity out of its massed cells? That Honey-eater is the deep principle of unity within, the One Life of all our lives, "near at hand" because the base and ground of all experience whatsoever. That One Life or *Ātman* is the Queen Bee, hidden in the hive, she whose presence gives unity to the scattered bees. Therefore is the *Ātman* said to be the Lord of past and future, for indeed all that has been and all that will be is held as a pattern in its all-embracing Light.

He who has seen that *Ātman*, has recognised that ultimate principle of unity, shrinks no more from any thing for he knows that nothing can disturb its peace and bliss. The seeming chaos of the outer life becomes for him a divinely ordered cosmos and he shrinks from nothing for he knows that in it everything has its place. Within him, Life of his life, Soul of his soul, is the Deathless being whose vision ranges through eternities, the stainless Immortal One, the divine Sphinx whose calm eyes gaze forever over the sands of Time. Those Eyes that saw the fall of lost Atlantis are gazing through our own eyes at this moment: those Ears that heard the thunder of the chariots at Kurukshetra are listening through our own ears even now.

It is only our false personal selves that, with their craving for separate existence, see not and hear not because of their separateness. Willingly immured in the prison cell of self, we complain that nothing is visible

193

save through the small barred window of the present
If we emerge from that cell, sinking our separate self ir
That which is its true Reality and Ground, the wide-
extended earth and all the blue infinities of heaven li
open to our gaze. No more need we long for the friend's
face to pass our little window, no more grieve wher
he has gone beyond and out of sight. Wherever he is
our now unfettered sight can be with him, for never car
he or anything pass beyond the edges of that Plain o:
Truth which now extends unbroken before our gaze
the Plain which, like the high plateaux of central Asia
offers no obstacle to the free-ranging Soul.

Such is the vision of the Deathless One within us
he who is our very Self. As we approach His Being
we may know it by the fact that the prison walls grov
thin and unsubstantial, so that, as through a thinning
mist we see the landscape, so through the mists of time
ages long dead and ages yet unborn blend into on
great pattern of which the present is but the focal point
"A thousand years are but a day" in the vision of th
Ātman and by this characteristic we may recognise Hi
nearness. This verily is That.

Before leaving this verse we must note that it
concluding words *tato na vijugupsate* which, followin;
Shankara, have been rendered as 'thereafter he shrink
away no more' are susceptible of another and a deepe
interpretation. They may equally well be translated a
'from that (Ruling Power) he shrinks away no more.
At first sight such an interpretation may come as rathe
a shock and, in fact, seem almost without meaning
We are used to the idea that men, at least men who con
cern themselves with such texts at all, are engaged i
seeking, with more or less of strenuousness, for 'Goc
or the *Ātman* and we may well wonder why it shoul
be stated that at a certain stage the disciple will shrin
away from Him (or It) no more.

Nevertheless it is so. Far from seeking 'God' most men, even most 'religious' men, spend their time in avoiding and hiding from Him. Not for nothing does the Bible call God a 'consuming Fire,' a thought which will be taken up in the next few verses of our text. Our present verse has already referred to the *Atman* as the Ruler of Past and Future, or in other words, as the Lord of Fate, and we have seen that what we term Fate is the compulsion which arises from those parts of our psyche that are hidden from the consciousness of the ego. It is thus in very truth the *Atman* who, as the Hound of Heaven, pursues us "down the arches of the years," and it is to protect the idolised ego from the consuming fires of that *Atman* that we erect all sorts of barriers, the barrier of social convention, the barrier of science and philosophy, the barrier of a religious creed, anything in fact that will serve to ensure that the daemonic and elemental Powers of the universe, inner or outer (and they are the same), the Power of Fate in short, shall only impinge upon the ego after being tamed or disinfected by having to pass through the 'recognised channels.' This is the reason why the bureaucrat erects a fence of red tape around himself, society, a wall of conventions, the materialist, one of scientific dogma and the exoterically religious man a protective creed which will bar out all daemonic visitants except such as bring with them the certificate of orthodoxy.

As we have said before, the path to the *Atman* is the Path of Death, a Path that begins and ends in Fire; it is no wonder that the ego shrinks away with all its childish might and seeks to hide its head under the bed clothes of use and wont.

It is true that the *Atman* is the Friend of all beings; nevertheless, on the authority of the Gita[1] and by the

---

[1] Gita, VI, 5, 6.

testimony of plain fact, it can and often does pursue us with the fury of relentless Fate, Artemis the Huntress urging on her hounds in pursuit of the rash mortal who, unpurified, has entered her dark and sacred forest. Therefore it is that between us and that forest is erected a wall beyond which we do not venture, though in it we erect a shrine at which we may pay decorous worship to the Power we fear to face. Most talk of the 'merciful and loving Heavenly Father' is precisely of this sort, for now, as in the ancient world, names are reassuring and the blankets of euphemism hide our heads from forms we fear to see. Thus did the *Erinyes*, the Terrible Ones, become the Gracious *Eumenides*.

The truth is that to the *unpurified* ego the *Brahman* or *Ātman* is a terrible figure and it is as such, indeed, in the form of a *Yaksha* that it appears to the Gods in *Kena Upanishad*. Most of us spend all our lives in the safety of the city and rely on a variety of watchmen at the gates to protect us from all that is strange and which might therefore be a disguised form of the awesome and shape-changing Dragon who dwells in the forests outside the walls. The Initiate is one who has left the walls behind him, who has braved the perils of the unknown, who has met the Dragon face to face, and, overcoming him, has bathed in his blood, thus becoming a Dragon himself.

For if the Dragon is the Devil, he is also God. The Flames that emerge from his nostrils are death to the coward ego but they are also the sacred Fire of rebirth, the Nachiketas Fire in fact, for the heroic Soul. Therefore in ancient writings the initiates were termed Dragons of Wisdom, and therefore, also, it was that, in the interests of the uninitiated many, rather than as often thought, because of the jealousy of the initiated few, the Gates of Initiation in Greece bore the inscription: "Flee far from here, O profane."

Chapter IV

To pass those Gates is death to the unpurified ego
which clings to its limitations and would remain forever fixed in its present one-sidedness. Only he who
would lose his life to find it, he who is content that the
shell of his self-hood should be dissolved in order
that the Phoenix of Self may rise in radiance from its
ashes, only he should venture through them. It is of
such that the text speaks when it affirms that he shrinks
away no more from the mysterious and awe-inspiring
Power which he has hitherto known as Fate, the two-
formed Dragon which he now knows to be the Life
of all beings, the Power at the heart of all manifestation, that which to every being whatsoever is the dearest
thing of all. This verily is That.

(6) *He who in the beginning was born from the inner
Heat* (tapas); *who was born earlier than the Waters*[1], *who,
having entered the Cave, stands; who gazed forth through beings
—-This verily is That.*

(7) *She who is manifested together with Life* (prāna)[2]
Aditi, *whose substance is the Gods, who, having entered
the Cave, stands; who was born forth distributively through
beings—This verily is That.*

(8) Agni, *Knower of Births, concealed in the two Fire
Sticks like the embryo well nourished by pregnant women,
worthy of daily worship from awakened·men who offer sacrifice—
This verily is That.*

(9) *Whence also the Sun rises and where it sets: on that
are established all the Gods. Truly none can pass beyond
it—This verily is That.*

In these verses we have a description of the One

[1] It can also be translated: "in the beginning was born from
the Waters."
[2] We can also translate: by Life. Some corruption of the
text has been suspected in both these verses.

Reality as divided into the three great cosmological Principles, the Trinity of Father, Mother and Son that has been worshipped in one form or another in most religions.

The first verse describes the Father or *Puruṣha*, the Light of transcendent Self-hood, the *Shānta Ātman* who is the beginning of manifestation, or rather who, before all actual manifestation, was born of the inner Heat of self-limitation. We have stated that in the ultimate Darkness of the *Parabrahman* there are two great Poles between which forever moves that ceaseless and mysterious Breath, ceaseless even in the Night of *Pralaya.* As the Dawn approaches it is as if the Light of Spirit or pure consciring that was, as it were, diffused through the Whole, concentrated itself at the central Pole, the Pole that is known as *Puruṣha* or the Sun. It is this concentration in a centre that is known as *tapas*, the cosmic analogue of what takes place in the heart of a yogi and consequently known by the same term. The Light is, so to say, withdrawn from the Whole and concentrated at the mystic Centre, whence it flashes forth as transcendent Self-hood, the Light of the *Ātman*, the basis of all subjectivity whatsoever.

There is an ambiguity in the reference to the Waters for, as stated in a foot note, the phrase can equally well be translated "in the beginning was born from the Waters." Nevertheless the difference does not amount to much in reality as the term Waters will have a slightly different reference in each case. In this second alternative the Waters would refer to the dark Matrix in which the Light was diffused and from out of which it crystallised at the Centre. Alternatively, adopting our first version, the Waters are the Great Mother, the *Mūlaprakṛiti* which is that aspect of the *Parabrahman* which, so to speak, remains when the Light is withdrawn to the centre. From this point of view the Birth of the

Chapter IV

Light is at least logically prior to the manifestation of the Waters. In any case we must not attempt too fine a logic in these transcendent Realms. The symbols should be allowed to unfold their own meaning naturally rather than be pressed too rigidly into mental categories.

The second verse (verse 7) deals with the Great Mother, the Boundless Waters of Space, She who is the Matrix out of which manifest all the Divine Powers that men know as Gods.[1] *Aditi*, literally the Unbounded, represents the other Pole, the great *Mūlaprakriti* which is the transcendent Root of all objectivity, the Moon as opposed to the Sun, the Matrix out of which comes forth all objective manifestation. She is the Waters on whose face the Spirit of God moved in the account given in Genesis.[2] She is said to arise together with *Prāṇa* or Life because Her manifestating is really simultaneous with that of the *Purusha* who is Light and Life, the "Light which is the Life of men."[3] The two manifestations cannot be separated. The concentration of the Light means the manifestation of the Waters and vice versa. We can distinguish in thought, but in reality we are dealing with two aspects of one process rather than with two distinct stages.

These Two are referred to in the Gita as the beginningless pair[4] and from their interaction arises the Third, *Agni*, the Son. First of all, however, we should note that both Father and Mother are said to enter into the Cave and to stand or dwell therein. Primarily, that Cave is the great Abyss of Outwardness in which

[1] Compare the words of Agrippa: "They (Orpheus and Pythagoras) called those Divine Powers which are diffused in all things Gods." *Three Books on Occult Philosophy.*

[2] Genesis, I, 2.

[3] St. John, I, 4.

[4] Gita, 13, 19.

199

the universal manifestation takes place, but, as above so below, and from *our* inverted point of view, in which the outer seems to be the real, it is the Abyss of Inwardness, the Cave of the Heart to which we have referred so often and in which dwell the Divine Pair throughout the ages. Note, however, that, while the *Purusha* or Sun is said to gaze forth through all beings, the *Prakriti* or Moon is said to be manifested through them. This difference in phrase corresponds to the difference in their respective roles, for, while the *Purusha* is the Root of consciousness, of That which is aware of all things, That which gazes out from behind our eyes, the *Prakriti* is the unmanifest Root of all manifested content, the very stuff of which all forms are made. It should hardly be necessary to mention that, in terming it 'stuff,' nothing that *modern* philosophers would call matter or material is meant, no tiny billiard-ball atoms of any sort, however rarefied. If the words stuff and matter are retained here it is because the psyche (and the ancient wisdom) had claims upon them long before our modern 'scientific' era. The true meanings of words must be sought in the eternal psyche and not in the ephemeral text books of science. The Tree of *Mūla-prakriti* and all its derivative branches is in a very real sense "such stuff as dreams are made on" and it is in that sense that the word is used. Let those who would understand its nature seek out that of which are composed the fleeting images of dream for the Dreaming State has well been called the Hall of Learning.

We should also note that both these principles, the *Purusha* and the *Prakriti*, the eternal Father and Mother are equated with the One Reality, the ultimate *Para-brahman* which the text refers to as That. They are identical with It because they are the two moments or Poles of its being. Apart from It and apart from each other, neither of them has any real or independent being.

Chapter IV

We now pass on to the Third Principle, referred to in verse 8, *Agni* the Fire, the Divine Son of the Two, concealed in their being like fire in the two fire-sticks which are their symbols. Just as the fire is born from the friction of the upper and lower fire-sticks, so does the Divine Agni flash forth from the interaction of the Divine Pair. He is "the Radiant Child of the Two, the unparalleled refulgent glory, Bright Space, Son of Dark Space, who emerges from the Depths of the great Dark Waters......He shines forth as the Sun, he is the blazing divine Dragon of Wisdom."[1] At least two hundred hymns in the Rig Veda sing his glories in his various forms for he is manifest upon all planes, and in his deepest being is identical with the unmanifest Black Fire of the one Reality. He is in fact the Ever-Living Fire of Heracleitus, the Fire which burns in the heart of the Sun and in the heart of man. He is the Lord of the House, the Guest in every human Abode (i.e., in every body), the nearest Kinsman, the Wise Seer, the Producer of Wisdom, and, as the Ladder between Heaven and Earth, the messenger of the Gods.[2] Words fail to describe his glories as they also fail to express the exasperation felt at the triviality of academic 'explanations.'

He is that one Thing, "The Force of all forces, that ascends from earth to heaven and descends again, new born, to earth."[3] "O Divine Shepherd, Sole Seer, Controlling power, O sun, O child of *Prajāpati*, expand thy Rays and concentrate the splendour of thy heart. That Form which is the fairest of all forms, that Form of thine I see."[4]

---

[1] *Stanzas of Dzyan.*
[2] All these are common Vedik epithets of Agni.
[3] *The Smaragdine Tablet.*
[4] *Ishopanishad,* 16. This prayer is no doubt addressed to the

He burns in Earth and Air and Water; he burns in the heart of man and beast; he burns in sun and stars and, most wonderful of all, in the Black Space that is beyond all stars. From the Dark Waters he flashes forth in birth and yet he is the Power which holds those Waters in its grasp. He is both Son and Father of his Parents, the radiant Child of Dawn, the hidden Lord of Night. He is the Knower of Births for it is He himself who, in a thousand forms, is born in all that is. Moreover, he who knows the Fire knows all that is, the secret of all being, nor is there any form which at his will he cannot transmute to any other, for he himself becomes Knower of Births, a Maker of all forms. Wherever there is form, there, in its hidden heart, flames the Divine *Agni*. All things he burns to ashes and yet all he makes anew in golden tongues of fire. All Gods are forms of Him though He is form of Nought. Assuredly there is none more worthy of "daily worship from those who are awakened."

"That which is Flaming, subtler than the subtle; on which the Worlds are fixed with all their dwellers; That is the Imperishable Brahman."[1]

From Him the Sun arises in the morning; by Him his chariot soars through the mid-heaven and into Him again he sinks at Night. All the worlds are but the declension of Fire: beyond it there is Nothing. "You will enter the light but you will never touch the Flame." This verily is That.

> (10) *Whatever is here, that is there;*
> *Whatever is There, that also is here;*
> *From death to death he goes,*
> *Who sees things here as different.*

Sun but the latter is but the highest form of *Agni* manifest upon this physical plane of experience.

[1] *Muṇḍaka Upanishad*, 2, 2, 2.

Chapter IV

(11) *By the* manas *indeed is this to be realised;*
     There is not even the slightest difference here.
     From death to death he goes
     Who sees things here as different.

We now come to one of the central teachings that
are inscribed on the Inner Door, the teaching known in
the West as the Hermetic Axiom and given in the celebrated Emerald Tablet as follows:—

"It is true, certain and without falsehood, that whatever is below is like that which is above; and that which
is above is like that which is below: to accomplish the
one Wonderful Work."

This teaching is to be found in all the mystical
schools. Thus Plotinus tells us that "all that is Yonder
is also Here" and the Kabalistic tradition of the Zohar
affirms that "esoterically the man below corresponds
entirely to the Man Above."[1]

There are those who have not yet found the Inner
Door and who will be disposed to question the application of the term axiom to this teaching. Some will call
it mere analogy (and perhaps a dubious analogy) while
others will consider that it would be better to call it
a postulate of occult philosophy rather than an axiom.
Nevertheless the fact remains that for those who have
found that Door it *is* an axiom, *the* axiom in fact, upon
which the Hidden Science is built. To him who reaches
that Door its truth is as self-evident as is the statement
that two and two makes four.

We have already referred to the fact that the
manifested universe can be divided into two great

---

[1] There is also a version in the Tantrik tradition (*Vishvasara
Tantra*): "Whatever is here is Elsewhere, what is not here is nowhere at all." One may also add that the sentence in the Lord's
Prayer "Thy will be done on earth as in heaven" has the same
meaning.

Spheres or Hemispheres of being which may be called the Above and Below and which are symbolised by the Celestial and Terrestrial Spheres. These two Spheres are in complete correspondence with each other and that for the very simple reason that the Lower is the reflection of the Upper. Every movement of the Stars is reflected down here on Earth and it is through the study of experience here that we are able to advance to an understanding of the archetypal structure of experience 'yonder.'

On all planes and sub-planes of the Cosmos this Axiom rules. It is the master-key which will open all locks. The mere possession of the key as an intellectual doctrine will no doubt lead to all sorts of merely analogical reasoning which may lead the enquirer nowhere in particular; but the image of the key printed on the pages of a book is not the Key and our statement applies solely to him who has found the Key itself. For him the four great Doors that are at the four cardinal points of the Cave of Initiation stand open, Doors that are symbolised in all the temples of India and which will give him entry into strange and secret passages that lead to all the Quarters of the universe. There is a sacred cavern in the Himalayas from which underground passages are popularly supposed to go to far-off Benares and Prayag. The actual passages are probably a myth; nevertheless the symbolism is true, though the mystic cities to which they lead are not the ones bearing the same names that can be reached by rail.

"By the *manas* is this to be realised," or, translating more literally, 'obtained.' The reason for this statement becomes evident when we consider the central position of *manas*, the point of intersection between the upper and lower triangles. It is the point-like window through which the Above is reflected as the Below and also the Door which leads from one Hemisphere into the other.

To translate *manas* by that hold-all English word 'mind' is to risk complete misunderstanding and to substitute for the real Key that will unlock the secret passages a brown paper cut-out that will collapse into pulp at the first shower.

The teaching that the Axiom is to be gained by the *manas* most assuredly does not mean that it is just to be thought about or made the centre of a lot of intellectual speculations. The gaining of the Axiom refers to a real process, namely, that of transferring the heart conscious-ness from the false, one-sided centre of the personal self to the true centre or higher Self.

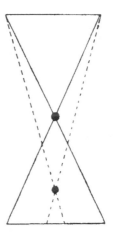

The above diagram should make it quite clear. Under all conditions the above is reflected in the below through the *mānasik* focus. If, however, that focus is in the lower *manas* the result, as shown by the dotted lines, is that the reflection is an unbalanced one, and, of the total range of experience that might be had down here, only a fraction is available to the mental conscious-

ness. It is thus that we perceive only a small fragment
of what we might perceive, all the rest being outside
the focus of the waking personal self. Moreover it will
easily be seen that the more one-sided, the 'lower,' the
further from the true Centre, our ordinary ego integration is placed, the more limited is our field of vision.
Truly we are blinded by our own one-sidedness. This
is why "the fool sees not the same tree that a wise man
sees."[1]

When we can learn to focus our being in the true
Centre of the Higher *manas* the world of perception down
here undergoes a great expansion. A great range of
experience previously hidden from us now becomes
manifest and now only is it seen that the Below reflects
the Above in perfect correspondence. This is the
gaining of the Axiom.

For one who has gained it there can be no more
question of states to be achieved after death, of ranges of
being to be explored with the aid of supernormal trance
states, for all things are open to him here and now. In
the calm clear waters of the *Mānas* lake the Stars above
are perfectly reflected as the grasses of the field below,
and, to the eye of such a Seer, nowhere is there any
difference at all. Wherever he looks, Up or Down, he sees
the same Divine Harmony, the Harmony of "Heaven
above, Heaven beneath" and, having seen, he is happy.
Nor is this new vision of his in any sense a merely 'spiritual' one, using that word with the implications that it
has for the average man, namely, of something 'poetic,'
very beautiful, but not quite 'real.' It is an experience
that is entirely real, entirely practical. On it is based
the whole mighty structure of Occult Science, a science
that is infinitely more powerful and far-reaching than
the science of our day, one by which, as Hermes put

[1] Biake: *The Marriage of Heaven and Hell.*

it, "many rare wonders are wrought." Even true
Faith can, as Christ said, move mountains, and Faith,
as we have said, is but the reflection of Knowledge
not yet fully manifest or available. What then shall
be said of Knowledge in its fulness ? He who has known
the Axiom has the Key to all transformations whatsoever. Should he desire to do so he can transmute lead
into gold with as much ease as the common test-tube
chemist can produce copper out of copper sulphate, and
indeed, to quote Christ again, far greater things than
these can he accomplish "because I go unto my
Father."[1]

Such a one is indeed a *Siddha*, an Adept, Dragon of Wisdom, Master of Immortality, Lord of the
Double-Axe.

As for the ordinary man, he who still sees difference between Below and Above, between here and Here-
after, material and spiritual, he, in the words of the text,
goes from death to death. This is inevitable because
such unbalanced seeing is the vision of the lower or
false self and we have already pointed out how death
and again death is the inevitable result of any one-sidedness of integration. As long as we cannot see the Above
and the Below as one and the same, so long are we at a
distance from our true Centre and so long is the cycle
of birth, death and rebirth an inevitable one for us. As
the Buddha taught, so long as we identify our being
with the *attā*, the false self, so long are we bound upon
the ever-whirling Wheel. Only when we can see
things *yathā bhūtam*, as they really are, only then are we
free, for only then are we poised in the true Centre.

This brings us to the nature of that Centre of which

---

[1] St. John, 14, 12. These last words have of course a mystic
meaning which should be evident to him who has followed the
Upanishad thus far.

something is said in the next verses.

(12) *In the midst of our being* (ātmani) *stands the Dweller*[1] *of the size of thumb, the Lord of Past and Future. (He who has attained) shrinks away from Him no more. This verily is That.*
(13) *The Dweller of the size of a thumb is like Smoke-less Flame, Lord of the Past and Future, He alone Is To-day and He, To-morrow.*

The word *ātmani*, here translated as 'being' is of course literally 'self' but is explained by Shankara as meaning body. This is correct as far as it goes but it is only partial because what is really referred to is the centre of our whole psychic being which includes, but is by no means limited to, the physical body. On the level of that body, the centre is of course the heart but that heart is not *merely* the lump of flesh known by that name for it extends inwards in dimensions not known to modern scientific thought. It is, in fact, the true centre of our being and it is characteristic of our modern one-sidedness that most men nowadays feel themselves to be centred in the head, which most emphatically is not the true Centre, was not felt to be such by the ancients and is not so felt by yogis even now. The feeling of the self in the head is just that eccentricity or one-sidedness which we have been describing. He who lives in his head shall lose that head but he who lives in his heart shall stand forever.[2]
In the Heart, then, is the Dweller who has been described as of the size of a thumb and is indeed the

[1] *Purusha*, he who dwells in the *pura* or city.
[2] Perhaps it will be objected that it has just been said that the ancients lived in the heart but they have not 'stood for ever.' Never mind: it is quite true.

same small but mighty being who is known in Western myth as Tom Thumb. He is also the celebrated Homunculus or Little Man, the creation of whom was one of the objects of alchemists such as Paracelsus. Popular belief represented him as being created in a bottle but in truth the unique vessel in which he is born is not a glass but a Golden one made of the famous Gold of the Philosophers, true Gold but perfectly transparent.

He is the Man-Child which the Woman brought forth, as described in the Book of Revelations,[1] the Child which the Dragon sought to devour, but who is destined to "rule all nations with a Rod of Iron." He is born in the Fire and the *Secret of the Golden Flower* informs us that "a whole year of this Fire-period is needed before the Embryo is born, sheds the membranes and passes out of the ordinary world into the holy world."

Who is this mysterious Child and what is the meaning of his Birth? The first question is easily answered. He is the Inner Ruler and the Rod of Iron with which he rules is a definite fact. "From the most ancient times till to-day, this is not empty talk."[2] He is the Central Point, the Focus to which we have so often referred, and as such is essentially Unborn. The *Maitri Upanishad*[3] describes his being as two-fold, as being a Light of two-fold or three-fold brightness and in another place[4] we read that when manifesting the qualities of *Atma* and *Buddhi* only he is "like the point of an awl" in size, a mere focal point through which the Sunlight of the *Atman* streams forth. On the other hand, when united with the formative and ego-producing *manas* (*sankalpa ahankāra samanvita*) he manifests as the Smokeless Flame of the

---

[1] *Revelation* 12, 4 and 5.
[2] *The Secret of the Golden Flower.*
[3] *Maitri Upanishad* 6. 38.
[4] *Shwetāshwatara Upanishad* 5. 8.

14

Thumb-like *Purusha* and it is this manifestation that is referred to as his Birth. The same Upanishad teaches that he is manifested by means of the mind, the *Buddhi* and the Heart, and that they who know Him become immortal, words which find an echo in the Chinese text which tells us that "if this method of ennobling is not applied, how will the way of being born and dying be escaped ?"

The actual Birth is brought about by the application of the old alchemical formula, *solve et coagula*. First comes the Fire-period in which the one-sided integration of the ordinary Self, the lower *manas*, has to be melted by the help of the Nachiketas Fire in the Unique Vessel already referred to. "Not till the whole personality of the man is dissolved and melted—not until it is held by the divine fragment which has created it, as a mere subject for grave experiment and experience— not until the whole nature has yielded and become subject to its higher Self, can the Bloom open."[1] In other words, only when the dissolving process is complete and the false self is dead can the second stage, the Birth or crystallising out of the new Form be commenced. The alchemists termed this a sublimation for it is a process by which the essence of the Death's Head, the dark matrix into which the lower principles have been dissolved, are caused to ascend to the upper portions of the Vessel where, under the formative rays of the Stars above, they crystallise out into the living Form of the Golden Flower, the Thumb-like *Purusha*, the Smokeless Flame, the deathless Lord of Time. He is of course what is often termed the higher Ego but "how empty, stale, flat and unprofitable" seems all this modern language of the mind with its all-explaining

---

[1] *Light on the Path.* The 'divine fragment' is of course the Centre itself, small as the "point of an awl."

pride and its spurious, sterile clarity. Shall a man love and worship a 'higher Ego' and without love how shall there be birth ? Not in the glass-cases of our dead and damnable museums, not amidst the pale ghosts of our abstract thought is He to be found, but in the mystic darkness of the ancient temples, whose outer walls are covered from top to bottom with the rich symbols of the eternal Soul.

He is the Thumb of power, and of creative manifestation, the fiery Will that is the heart of Man. He is the youthful *Kārtikeya*, the glorious Master of the Heavens, and, from one point of view at least, he is the four-faced *Brahmā* seated in the midst of the Dark Waters, enthroned upon the golden Lotus which springs from the very navel of the Sleeping Spirit who is their In-dweller. In Egypt he was known as Harpocrates, Horus the Child, he whose finger was ever on his lips in token of silence concerning the secret of his Birth from dead Osiris. He was also represented as the Look-out, seated at the prow of the Ship of the Soul and a lock of his hair was worn by the candidate for Initiation as a talisman which would serve to introduce him to the Gods.[1]

It is of this sacred Birth that we find Isis saying to her Son, Horus: "I may not tell the story of this Birth, for it is not permitted to describe the origin of thy Descent, O Horus, son of mighty power, lest afterwards the way-of-birth of the immortal Gods should be known unto men."[2] In truth the secret is safe enough for it is

[1] The symbolism of this may perhaps be more easily understood with the help of a quotation from Hermes. "Who then doth have a Ray shining upon him through the Sun within his rational part—and these in all are few—on them the Daimons do not act; for no one of the Daimons or of Gods has any power against one Ray of God." *Definitions of Asclepius.*

[2] *The Virgin of the World*, I, 36.

one that cannot be put into words and as Hermes says: "This Race, my son, is never taught; but when He willeth it, its Memory is restored by God......I can but tell thee this. Whenever I see within myself the Un-compounded Vision[1] brought to birth out of God's mercy, I have passed through myself into a Body that can never die. And now I am not what I was before; but I am born in Mind. The way to do this is not taught and it cannot be seen by the compounded element by means of which thou seest."[2]

At any rate sufficient has been said to indicate the nature of this *Puruṣha* or Dweller in the Heart. On account of his Central position he is the Lord of Fate which arises as we have said from that which is 'behind' one. For him, with eyes on every side, there is no 'behind' and before and therefore no Fate. He is the One-whose-Hour-shall-never-strike; he is beyond the Cycles; time's flow as known to us has ceased for him and past and future blend in one Eternal Present.

He verily is That.[3]

(14) *As water rained on a high peak runs away amongst the hills, so he who sees objects*[4] *as separate runs away in pursuit of them.*

(15) *As pure water poured into pure water becomes the*

---

[1] Compare the Uncompounded Element (*asanskṛita dhātu*) of the Buddhists.

[2] Hermetic Corpus XIII, 2 and 3.

[3] The last line in verse 12 has the same double sense as in verse 5. There is no need to repeat what was said there.

[4] *dharmān*: sometimes translated as 'qualities' but really meaning, elements of experience, especially sensory experience. Thus the experience of redness is a *dharma*. What we call objects are in reality patterns of such *dharmāḥ*. The word was much used in this sense by the Buddhists and also by Gauḍapada in his *Māṇḍūkya Kārikas*.

Chapter IV

*very same, so, O Nachiketas, becomes the Self of the Wise
seer.*

In these two verses the Way of death and the Way
of life are taught respectively. The first is the path
trodden by the ordinary man, he who sees himself as a
separate entity (the central mountain) surrounded by a
world of separate objects, the surrounding hills. The
Water of Life which descends upon him runs down in
all directions and is lost among those hills. "The
force of the Light exhausts itself and trickles away......
Take heed! If for a day you do not practise meditation,
this Light streams out, who knows whither." Thus
"the primordial Spirit is scattered and wasted. When
it is completely worn out, the body dies."[1] Each time
we pursue outside ourself that which is only to be found
within us we waste that Light. Identifying ourselves with transient patterns we share their transiency
and die with them. For this reason the Sages have always taught that we should restrain the Heart-Light
from flowing out towards objects but should let it remain collected in the Heart like the clear mirror of a
mountain lake. When this is done, the entire Cosmos
is mirrored in the serene waters; all things are seen
to be within the Self; pure water has been poured into
pure water and runs nowhere but remains the same.
The outflow of desire has ceased for ever. Therefore it
has been said: "The seed-blossom (i. e., the Light)
of the human body must be concentrated upward in the
empty space. Immortality is contained in this sentence and also the overcoming of this world is contained
in it. That is the common goal of all religions".[2]

[1] *The Secret of the Golden Flower.*
[2] *Ibid.*

CHAPTER V

(1) *Watching over[1] the eleven-gated City of that birth-less undistorted Consciousness one grieves not, and, when liberated (from the body), is freed indeed.*
This verily is That.

The eleven-gated City is of course the city of the Psyche, what Bunyan termed the City of Mansoul. Not only is it that in which the Psyche dwells, it is also the Fortress which the latter has built up in order to preserve its own separate individuality and to fence itself off from a hostile outer world. To identify it, as is sometimes done, with the physical body is to take a part for the whole. The City is surrounded by several Walls and the physical body is only the outermost of them all, and included within that outer rampart is much that is not physical at all.

The eleven gates are the eleven senses by which the outer world enters in and through which the Dweller in the body sallies forth to act upon that world.[2] Hindu philosophy, as is well known, classifies the senses into five organs of knowledge, hearing, seeing, touching, tasting and smelling; five organs of action, speaking, locomotion, handling, excreting and procreating, together with the (lower) *manas* as the eleventh, synthe-

[1] *Anushthāya*, literally, standing by.
[2] Some translators explain these eleven gates as the eleven bodily orifices, seven facial ones, the suture in the top of the skull, the navel and the two lower ones. In a secondary sense, possibly; but it is not by watching over one's navel or sagittal suture that one is freed from sorrow.

sising or 'common' sense. These are the eleven gates of access to or from the City of the Soul, and, with the exception of certain trance states, at all times traffic is passing through them to and fro. Even during sleep when the outer or gross senses are inactive, their subtle inner counterparts are, except in the state of deep sleep (*sushupti*), still in operation.

If a man is to live he must eat and therefore it behoves him, if he wishes to remain healthy, to be careful of what he eats. Similarly, the interplay between the psyche and its environment, the play of sense-life, is always going on and it is therefore necessary that we should watch over it carefully if the psyche is neither to be poisoned by what it takes in nor wrecked by the violent reactions caused by what it sends out. On the Path or off it, the sense-life must go on, "nor indeed can embodied beings completely abandon action."[1] The traffic through the Gates, however, can be restricted to what is essential and even that can and must be carefully scrutinised on its way out and in. This is the process known to the Buddhists as right recollectedness, the only real way of mastering the sense-life. The Soul is like the captain of a ship, depending on the winds for his power of movement but forced to exercise an unremitting watchfulness night and day if he is to avoid being led astray or capsized by those same winds. "Seek (the Path) by testing all experience, by utilising the senses in order to understand the growth and meaning of individuality."[2] I speak, but what am I speaking and why ? This is the type of watchfulness that must be constantly exercised. Even in sleep a night watch must be kept—at least on the later stages of the Path— and we read of the Buddha that "calm and self-recol-

[1] *Gita* 18, II.
[2] *Light on the Path.*

lected" he lay down to sleep. Nor should we be content with mere superficial answers to the above questions. There are deep unseen currents that sway the thoughts and deeds of men. Even the passive perceptive life is moulded by them and we see, not merely what is 'in front of us', but a selection that has been largely determined by those unseen tides of desire which can on occasion even bring it about that we see what is not there and hear that which was never spoken. There are traitors in our City who seek to pass in and out under the guise of honest citizens and deep and searching must our enquiries be if we are to detect their hidden purposes. It is not just a question of 'is this that I am saying true?' The Devil can quote scripture for his ends and even a true statement can be used for purposes that are by no means in accordance with the *Ṛita* or Harmony. It is this accordance with the Harmony and not any mere text-book rules of ethics that must be the touchstone to which we bring all experience.

It will be asked whether all this self-examination is not liable to become a neurotic habit, one, moreover, which will dry up and sterilise the springs of action. Certainly it *can* become such and indeed often does. This is, as we have already been told, the Razor-edged Path, and those who are frightened by its dangers had better leave it alone. Dangerous or not, it is the only method (except perhaps one of which we shall not speak here and in which it is really also included) by which the sense-life may be mastered and brought under control.

The Path can never be foolproof, still less can it be proof against the deliberate mischief of that jigging ape, the lower mind, if the Soul chooses to identify itself with it. Incidentally we should not forget that that particular ape is very definitely one of the eleven which have to be watched, in fact the chief of the eleven, only too often their Judas Iscariot, he who has the

bag. Nevertheless there is a safeguard that is mentioned in the text. The real Consciousness of the Soul is
stated to be *avakra*, not bent, or, as we have translated,
not distorted. We need not repeat the explanations
already given of how the one-sided integration of the
lower self produces a strain which results in the distortion of all the psychic processes, thus bringing it
about that our ordinary consciousness is *vakra*, bent
or distorted by the stresses of desire. If it is of such
distorted consciousness that our watchmen are composed they will themselves betray us and nothing can save
our city from that civil strife which we nowadays term
neurosis. Before we can set about the process of
watching we must discover a body of honest citizens
from among whom to choose our watchmen. In
other words, before we can master the sense-life we
must first seek out and discover the Fount of pure and
undistorted consciousness that wells up in our hearts.
Even in the most unbalanced or neurotic of us that
Fount is forever sending up its pure and limpid waters.
In them we must bathe, not once but constantly, if we
are to achieve the mastery we seek. Only when gleaming wet with its purifying waters can we stand aside
in detachment from the distorted consciousness of the
lower personality and only then can we hope to "grasp
and guide it."[1] Then and not till then can we use all
its powers and devote them to a worthy service.

These Waters are our only safeguard. They and
only they can save our yoga from degenerating into that
over-conscientious scrupulosity which makes life a hell
for many 'religious' people and not only sicklies o'er
the native hue of resolution, but, more serious still,
dries up the healing springs of laughter. Once that
occurs disaster is certain. Laughter was given by the

[1] *Light on the Path.*

Gods to man and it was one of their choicest gifts. No animal can laugh, nor does it need to since it lives in the harmony of the purely instinctive life. It is only Man whose possession of an ego introduces stresses and strains which cannot be avoided and for the healing of which, therefore, the Gods gave him this supreme gift. Time and again it will save us when otherwise all would be lost. He who cannot laugh, he whose devotions are too serious for the healing waves of laughter, had better look out: there are breakers ahead![1]

To return, however, to our text. If we can clothe ourselves with those waters of the pure consciousness we shall find that we are able to keep watch upon the coming and going of the sense-life not only without losing our balance but with a new and keen insight that will penetrate far below the surface pretensions of those who come and go.[2]

Mere ascetic suppression of the senses is impossible and the attempt highly dangerous. The outer senses may be forcibly controlled by the will but such violent repression only drives their activity inwards and their twin brothers, the inner senses, then run riot in a welter of fantasy which is far more harmful to the health of the psyche and far more destructive of yoga than any outer sense activity could possibly be. "He who sits controlling the organs of action but dwelling in his mind

---

[1] Laughter supplies the best medicine for *sacroids*. A sacroid may be defined as a hard morbid growth (sometimes becoming malignant) composed of a particular type of holy matter very sensitive and too sacred to be touched. They usually occur in the head. They are however not "the precious jewel in the head" which they are often mistaken for, and, as they greatly interfere with the freedom of the life-breath, they should be dissolved at once, without delay.

[2] Compare the twin processes known to Buddhists as *Shamathā* and *Vipashyana*, usually translated calm and insight. The Waters are the calm; insight the result.

on the subtle objects of the senses, that deluded man is called a hypocrite."[1]

What is required is not repression but watchfulness, through watchfulness understanding and through understanding control. The disciple must (robed always in the Waters) watch the activities of his senses and understand *why* they seek to act as they do and what results follow from such action. On this point the teachings of the Buddha are quite clear: "When, in following after happiness or after sense objects, I have perceived that bad qualities developed and good qualities were diminished, then I have considered that that happiness or those sense objects are to be avoided, while, when I have seen that the reverse is true, I have considered them as fit to be followed after."[2] Having watched in this way the disciple will find himself able to understand the sense life, inner as well as outer, and, having understood, he will be in a position for the first time to master it, to rule it with the iron rod of a mind that is united to and controlled by the eternal harmony of the *Buddhi* which it reflects.

Thus indeed one passes beyond sorrow and, when liberated from the body which is the crystallisation or precipitate of all our previous unbalanced actions, no forces remain to bring about the formation of a new one.

> "He—dying—leaveth as the sum of him
> A life-count closed, whose ills are dead and quit,
> Whose good is quick and mighty, far and near.
> So that fruits follow it.
> No need hath such to live as ye name life.
> That which began in him when he began

---

[1] *Gita* 3. 6.
[2] *Digha Nikāya* 21 (somewhat abridged).

Is finished: he hath wrought the purpose through
Of what did make him Man."[2]

Nevertheless, "The great and difficult victory, the
conquering of the desires of the individual soul, is a
work of ages; therefore expect not to obtain its reward
until ages of experience have been accumulated."

(2) (*He exists as*) *the Swan in the Clear, as the Pervader* (*Vasu*) *in the Mid-Space, as the Priest on the Altar
and as the Guest in the Sacred Jar;* (*He is*) *in Man, in the Superior* (*beings*), *in the Harmony* (rita), *in the Sky.* (*He is*)
born in the Waters, *the* (*heavenly*) *Cows, the Sacrifice* (*or
Harmony,* rita) *in the Sacred Stones.* (*He is*) *the Harmony*
(rita), *the Great one.*

This verse is a quotation from the Rig Veda and
its correct translation is to some extent conjectural as
the symbolic terms have, like so many Sanskrit words,
many alternative meanings. Nevertheless certain things
stand out clearly.

In the first place the verse occurs in a hymn to
Dadhikrāvana, the great Winged Stallion who "bounds
along the curves of the Paths." His name means the
Scatterer of the Curds and these two facts alone will
suffice to indicate what it is that he symbolises, especially if we add that he is most closely connected with *Ushas*,
the Dawn.[2] Readers of the Stanzas of Dzyan will remember Fohat who is the Steed of which "Thought is
the Rider," Fohat who also runs "on circular errands."

---

[1] *Light of Asia.*
[2] The academics of course have their own way of looking at
him. He is either some aspect of the sun which scatters the curds
of dew or frost at dawn or, alternatively, he is a deified race horse
who bounded along the curved paths of some ancient Aryan race
track.

They will also remember the Milk-white Curds which "spread throughout the depths of the Mother" and which were scattered through Space by the power referred to as Fohat at the time of the Cosmic Dawn.

The great Winged Stallion to which the verse refers is in fact the mighty Power which wields the manifested universe, the great dynamism which throbs at the heart of all being. It may well be "connected with the Sun" as it is in truth the great Power which holds the sun and the other heavenly bodies on their circular paths. It is also the Power which shapes what astronomers term spiral nebulae, but, to forestall misunderstanding, it may as well be said at once that the nebulae are not the Curds or at least are only their reflection on this physical plane. Nevertheless, as above, so below; the contemplation of the tremendous forces that wield the inconceivably vast nebulae and scatter them in all directions through space at that universal dawn of concentrated energy which even scientists are forced to admit,[1] will serve to give some idea of the splendour of the great Stallion as he rushes along the "curved paths."

"Verily the Dawn is the head of the Sacrificial Horse, the Sun his eye, the Air its life-breath, the Universal Fire its open mouth, the great Time Cycle is its body. The heavens are its back, the Mid-Space its belly, the Earth its hoofs, the Cardinal points its sides and the Intermediate Quarters its ribs, the Seasons its limbs, the Months and Fortnights its joints, the Days and Nights its feet, the Stars its bones, the Clouds its flesh......The Great Golden Vessel which appeared in front of the Horse is the Day. Its Source is the Eastern Sea. The Great Silver Vessel which appeared behind the Horse is the Night, its Source is the Western Sea. These two

---

[1] e. g., Eddington '*The Nature of the Physical World*' and other books.

arose on both sides of the Horse, as the two sacrificial Vessels. The Sea is indeed its Kinsman, The Sea its Source."[1]

He is the great Black Stallion with the Stars of heaven in his mane, the central Black Fire that burns at the Cosmic Heart, the Fire whose colour changes as it sweeps through all the worlds. Between the Sun and Moon he springs into manifest being, with their Birth he is born, and, as they separate, he bursts forth from the blackness at the heart of Space like a great jet of many-coloured Flame, the Fire of which the alchemists bid us "note the colours well," the Fire which so awed the great Arjuna on Kurukshetra's field:—

"I behold a sun-like blaze of fire crowned with the power of the Cycles, a mass of splendour in all the quarters of the Heavens, dazzling the gaze. Without beginning, middle, or end, infinite Power, the Sun and Moon thy eyes; I see Thy mouth, a blazing sacrificial Fire, consuming the universe with its heat!"[2]

This Fiery Stallion it is who is the Lord of Destiny for it is he who, born between Sun and Moon, controls the pattern that they weave upon the Wheel of Fate and it is for this reason that his various limbs are identified with the divisions of time.

The thunder of his great hooves as he gallops down the Rainbow Bridge of Space is heard echoing within the caverns of the heart like drums of doom. Therefore those caverns are a place of dread. Men turn and flee from that insistent drumming that haunts them, flee to the outermost regions of their being, into the delusive sunlight of the outer world where they plunge into the oblivion of a life of action or attempt to anchor

[1] *Brihadāranyaka Upanishad*, I, 1.
The two Vessels are of course the Sun and Moon.
[2] *Gita* VI 17 and 19.

their souls firmly to the material objects that surround them. But the attempt is a vain one, for all things, even the most solid and enduring, throb in tune with the Stallion's hoof-beats which called them into being and which dissolve them. As a glass whose note is sounded is shattered into a thousand tiny fragments, so the material things to which we cling disintegrate before our eyes and leave us with nothing that can distract our thoughts from the trampling hooves of That which follows. Few indeed are those who dare to turn and face the bloodshot eyes, to breathe the calm breath of power into the flaming nostrils, and, laying hand upon the star besprinkled mane, leap in the saddle and master thus their Fate. Such are the yogis, they to whom the Teacher speaks.

It will be wondered what all this has to do with the actual subject matter of the text. Our wanderings with the Heavenly Stallion, however, have not led us astray for we may remember that the Thumb-like *Purusha*, to which the next verse will return, was also described as the Lord of Fate and is indeed one of the Stallion's forms. For the latter is essentially the central Power, that which manifests through the Centre between the two Poles. The Stallion is born between the Sun and Moon, the Fire between the two-Fire-sticks and the Thumb-like Purusha manifests between the two halves of man's being, for he is, as we have said, a manifestation of the central Point, the higher *manas* and he dwells in the heart centre of the body. It is always and on all planes, through that Central Point that Power manifests because Power is in reality the fundamental Unity of being. Wherever two Poles come into manifestation, there the original and underlying Unity also manifests as a tension between them and it is that tension that we know as Power. Thus all life is, as Heracleitus taught, a play of opposites. All things are linked to their opposites by the unity out of which both are differentiated and it is that linkage which is responsible for the tendency all are subject to of passing into their opposites. Thus arises the incessant motion of the universe and all that is in it and it is this motion or the unity which causes it that we know as Power. Power is thus the ultimate *Parabrāhmik* Unity itself, a Unity which manifests upon all planes of the cosmos, the Seven and again the Forty-nine Fires of the Vedik tradition.

Our present verse enumerates four such Births, corresponding to the well-known four-fold division of the Cosmos into the states of *Jāgrat, Swapna, Sushupti,* and *Turīya.*

On the highest level, that of *Turīya,* it manifests as the mystic Swan, dwelling in the Clear Sky of transcendence and born of the Cosmic Waters. Its two wings are the Sun and Moon and the *Nādabindu Upanishad* tells us that "the adept who bestrides the Swan is not affected by the power of Karma." If, as is sometimes done, the Swan is identified with the Sun it is not the Sun as opposed to the Moon but rather the Sun as the Central Point of our system, that around which all revolves, the source of all Life and motion.

On the next level it manifests as the Pervading Power, the *Vasu* which dwells in the wide extended Mid-Space, the 'Superior.' The *Vasu,* which means the Pervader, is a name given to the Heavenly Gods, the Sky dwellers and there were said to be eight of such corresponding to the eight petals of the Mother Lotus, the *Prakṛiti.* The actual enumeration varies, but in the Vedik list, *Indra, Agni, Vishnu* and *Rudra* were all termed *Vasus.*[1] From the point of view of our present

[1] Later, under the influence of Pauranik theism the conception was altered somewhat and new lists are given excluding the

text the *Vasus* are the all-pervading Divine Powers that
dwell in the Great Space of the *Mahat*. Viewed as aspects of the Fire, they are tne Lightning which flashes
out in the central space between the clouds and it is for
this reason that they are said to be born of the (Heavenly)
Cows (*gojā*). In Indian art the clouds have always symbolised the ever-moving chariots of the Gods, and, as
the sources of the life-giving rain, they were also termed
the Heavenly Cows.

On the third level it manifests as the central Sacrificial Fire, *Agni*, known by Vedik Seers as the Priest,
because through him the offerings were transmitted
to the Gods. On this level it is said to dwell in the *Ṛita*
and to be born of the *Ṛita*. The *Ṛita* is primarily the
Cosmic Order, the Divine Harmony which governs all
things, that in which the very Gods have their being.
Secondarily, as that Order means the interlinkedness
and interdependence of all things as opposed to their
illusory separateness, it stands also for the sacrifice of
each for all and is the expression, real or symbolic, of
that interlinkedness. "Nourished by Sacrifice the Gods
bestow on you the objects of your desire. A thief is he
who enjoys their gifts without returning any."[1]

In this sense the Fire of the Sacrifice was the Power
which granted all gifts; of it the Lord of Beings had
said, "Be this to you the Giver of Desires,"[2] and therefore
in the Sacrifice the Power was born. Once more we
note that the Birth is a central one for it is the Fire which
is the intermediary between men and Gods. Moreover
it was from the friction of the two sacred Fire Sticks
that the Sacred Fire was made manifest; it was also the
central one among the five-fires maintained by the Brah-

greater Gods.
[1] *Gita* 3, 12.
[2] *Gita* 3, 10.

15

man householder. From the inner point of view it was the central Fire of *manas*, that to which the Fires of the senses transmitted their offerings, the Fire of Power that burns in their very midst.

Lastly, and on the lowest level, it is known as the Guest in the Sacred Jar, ritually a name that was given to the Soma Juice born between the two sacred Stones that were used to press it out (*adrija*). On this level he is said to be born in Man or in the world of men,[1] whose bodies are the real Jars in which he is the Guest. Just as the Swan was connected with the Sun, so is the Soma connected with the Moon.[2] The tawny-red juice as stored in the Jar (as opposed to the green unpressed plant) is the exhilarating Fire of Desire that courses through the veins of man, urging him to the accomplishment of actions from which at other times he would shrink. Here again the Lunar reference comes in, for the tides of Desire are swayed by the Moon and here too we have the central birth, for Desire is the intermediary between the *manas* above and the physical body below.

All these four Births are births of the one Universal Power and all are divine. In man the Swan may be said to hover above the head like the Solar Disk or the Divine Hawk in Egyptian sculptures or to be in the head itself in what the Tāntriks termed the Thousand Petalled Lotus. The *Vasu* is in the sixteen petalled lotus of the throat, the Priest in the centre known as the navel or solar plexus and the Soma in the loins. All are, however, the same Power that is centred in the

---

[1] It will be noticed that we have inverted the order of 'Man' and Sky in the second enumeration of the verse as the sense seems to require it, the three enumerations being clearly intended to be parallel. Note again the central birth between the two Stones.

[2] Soma and the Moon are identified symbolically and the word *atithi* or Guest is considered to be connected with *tithi* a lunar day.

Chapter V

Thumb-like *Purusha* in the Heart, the Cosmic creative Fire that is also the Fire of Doom.[1] It is the Great One, the *Ṛita*, for "this World-Order not man nor any of the Gods hath made but ever-living Fire kindled in measure and quenched in measure." Woe to him who seeks to misuse it for his selfish inharmonious purposes, whether on the level of the Soma, or on those higher levels unknown to the many. The higher the level, the more disastrous will be the consequences and for him it will be as a veritable Doom-Fire that it manifests.[2] For him, however, who can offer up all self in its flames, who can worship it as it burns on the sacrificial altar in the midst of the Cosmic Harmony, for him it will manifest as the beneficent divine Power, the Magic all-accomplishing creative Fire, Transmuter of all things, giver of Immortality.

(3) *The* Prāṇa *he leads upwards; in the opposite direction he casts the* Apāna; *He, the Dwarf seated in the Centre whom all the Gods sit near* (upāsate).[3]

(4) *Of the Embodied One, the Dweller in the body, on being loosed and freed from the body, what remains behind? This* (In-Dweller) *verily is That.*

(5) *Not by* Prāṇa *or* Apāna *does mortal ever live. By Another do men live, on which both these depend.*

The two terms *Prāṇa* and *Apāna* are often translated as the inbreath and outbreath. It is true that in some contexts they do have only this meaning but in reality the *Prāṇa* and *Apāna* are of much deeper significance.

---

[1] The *Kālānala of Gita* II, 25. It will be obvious that we are referring to the much talked of but little understood power known as *Kuṇḍalini Shakti*, "the mystic power that can make of thee a God."

[2] Such misuse being the essence of what is called black magic.

[3] The word also signifies worship.

Fundamentally they are the two great tidal movements of the Cosmos, the mysterious 'Breath' of the Breathless One referred to in the Rig Veda as 'breathing' even during the Night of Pralaya. In all things whatsoever this Breath, this rhythmic inflow and outflow, takes place perpetually. The Sun breathes, the earth breathes, the sea breathes, the very atoms breathe; all these breathings are the manifestations of the one great Breath. Where there is life there is breath and life is everywhere. Do not we even to this day speak of the living rock though we have come to think of it as a mere metaphor? Even the words used in the text indicate that something more than mere breath is being referred to, for 'upwards' is hardly the direction we should apply to the intake of air nor 'downwards' to our exhalations. Yet upwards, i.e., towards the Pole of Spirit, is the direction of the *Prāṇa* and downwards, towards the Pole of Matter, that of the *Apāna* and we have seen that on this physical plane the vertical polarity becomes a horizontal one. That which was upward in the Cosmos as whole becomes inward in man and that which was downward becomes outward.

These two great Cosmic tides, the movements in the directions of Spirit and Matter respectively, are, as we have said, reflected in all things whatsoever and not least in man, in whom they manifest in the breathing process. But this is only their most external manifestation. Man dwells simultaneously on many levels of being and each such level has its own appropriate 'breath.' It is for this reason that the *Haṭha yogi* lays so much stress on the practice of breath control (*prāṇāyama*). It is not the outer breath in itself whose control is so important to him but the subtle inner breaths, unperceived by the ordinary senses, but controllable through the control of the outer. The desire nature and the mind, for instance, have their own breaths and all these breaths are, like our ordinary breathing, manifestations of the one great Cosmic Rhythm. No wonder, then, that there are secrets hidden in the process of breathing. The normal respiratory rate, as doctors term it, is, for instance, connected with cosmic cycles of the utmost importance, though to go into this question would take us too far afield.

At least it should be clear that *Prāṇa* and *Apāna*, though including the processes of inhalation and ex-halation, really mean much more than these. What psychologists term introversion and extroversion, for instance, are only manifestations of these same two tidal movements. Again, when we passively receive a sensa-tion, the *Prāṇa* is operating, while, when we act upon the world, *Apāna* has come into play. The whole of life is indeed the interplay of their two movements. Health, physical or mental, is to be found in their correct balance, disease in their disharmony.[1] Hence again the *Haṭha yogi*'s use of breath-control for preserving or regaining health, a method, though, which, on account of its far-reaching but unseen effects, is highly dangerous except when taught by one with real knowledge.

What is it that controls these two all-regulating Tides in their ebb and flow? What indeed but the one Central Power which, as we have seen, is, on the microcosmic scale, the Thumb-like *Purusha*, seated in the centre, the Dwarf, small in stature but immense in power. He it is who is the real Breather. He breathes and all the bodily and mental functions breathe with him; he leaves

---

[1] The two great metabolic processes of the body, the building up and breaking down of cells, are entirely controlled by the *Prāṇa* and *Apāna*. In some places five great *Prāṇas*, *prāṇa*, *apāna*, *udāna*, *vyāna* and *samāna*, as well as hundreds of lesser ones are mentioned. Such classifications, however, are subsidiary ones, further differentiations of the two great 'Breaths' which, as referred to in our present text, divide the whole of life between them.

the body and all its breathing stops.

Not by mere inflow and outflow of air does man live. Such a flow can be maintained by artificial means, but, though it may serve to tide over a crisis, it cannot give life to a body which the in-dwelling Power, the mighty Dwarf, has abandoned. Truly, as the text says, it is not on the breath, nor even on the subtler inner breaths to which we have referred, that life depends but on 'Another,' the Breather. He sends his thought upward and we breathe in, downward and we breathe out. Around him are seated in their ordered ranks the hierarchies of the Sense and other living psychic Powers that the text refers to as the Gods, the Powers through whom the rich and varied world of experience is manifested in all its beauty and in all its terror. Those Powers *are* the Gods and all the ancient world knew them for such. It is only we moderns who, strutting pathetically on the ugly cast-iron balconies of the lower mind, look down in our fancied enlightenment and refer to Them as *only* sensations.

But they are not *only* anything and not all the ugly Latin words in our dictionaries are a sufficiently strong magic to destroy, though they may hide, their wonderful Divine being. Whatever we may say, all things are full of Gods, the ancient Gods through Whom were all things made that are made. The Sky is full of Gods, the Air, the Fire, the depths of Water and the broad expanse of Earth. And in each God are countless other Gods ranging from Heaven to Earth in dazzling hierarchies. In the blue of the sky, in the whiteness of the clouds, in the green of the fields, in the cool touch of deep waters, and the burning kiss of fire, in the sound of the wind, in the doomlike crack of the lightning, in the colour of flowers, in the song of birds, in the raging of the storm, yes and in the very shriek of tortured metal, are the Gods to whom these splendours owe their beauty or their terror. Everywhere, everywhere are Gods and nothing else; within us Gods, without us Gods; Gods of colour, Gods of sound, Gods of touch, and Gods of taste, Gods of the rushing surges of desire, Gods of the subtle movements of the mind. Gods of war, and Gods of peace, Gods of increase that bless the growing corn, Gods of decrease that rule in winter's death. Why endlessly enumerate ?—"All things are full of Gods."

The magic of the ancients was directed to the invocation of these Gods and their initiations were an introduction of the candidate to Their divine being, an unsealing of his eyes to Their beauty and power. "For you I call the glorious shining Agni, the Guest of men, whom all must strive to win even as a lover, God among Godly people, Knower of all Births. Sweet is his growth as of one's own possessions; his look when rushing forth to burn is lovely. He darts his tongue forth like a harnessed courser who shakes his flowing tail among the bushes. Like one athirst he lighteth up the forests; like water down the chariot ways he roareth. On his black path he shines in burning beauty, seen like the heaven that smiles through cloudy vapours."[1] We too have our magic, even our books of spells couched in long unintelligible words, but our magic is directed to the hiding of those same Gods and the initiations into our academic temples of knowledge, a process of learning to hide those Gods under the cloak of our Latin spells. No quotation is needed: any page of an encyclopaedia or scientific text book will suffice.

But it is not any polytheism (more learned magic !) that we are setting forth. These Gods, whether without or within the soul of man, are not a chaos of unrelated Powers but a cosmos united in the harmony of the Ṛita, that which governs all the cosmic movements and in

---

[1] *Rig Veda,* II, 4.

which all have their dwelling. They are also all arranged round the one Central Point of whose Power they are all manifestations, not the 'one true God', the abstract Monotheos of most modern religion, who is little else than a projection of the false ego upon a screen of clouds, but the Central Fire of the *Atman*, the Heavenly Stallion, the Mystic Dwarf who dwells in the heart of all beings. He it is who is the Pole-Star of the inner as of the outer Heavens, He who is surrounded by and worshipped by all the Gods. He it is whose presence in the body means its life and He whose departure causes it to fall apart in the chaos of death. When He departs nothing remains, the Nothing which is the Matrix out of which, at His coming, forms emerged, and into which, at His departure, they are resolved.

(6) *Now then I shall set forth to thee the Secret Eternal Brahman and also what happens to the Soul after death.*

(7) *Some Souls enter (again) a womb for re-embodiment; others go to the Fixed according to their* Karma *and according to their knowledge.*

There are two Paths that the Soul can follow after the death of the body which are known in other Upanishads as the Path of the Ancestors and the Path of the Gods respectively. The first leads through various stages to that heaven-world in which man reaps the fruit of his good deeds and thence back to incarnation in a human body. The second leads to the Fixed, the *Sthāṇu*, that which neither comes nor goes but remains firmly standing like a pillar of rock. That is the Path of Knowledge.

The word *Sthāṇu*, that which stands firm, is fixed, immoveable, a pillar, and is also a name of Shiva, has, as a secondary meaning, the pillar-like trunk of a tree, especially a branchless one. On the strength of that

fact many have interpreted the passage to the *Sthāṇu*
as reincarnation in the form of a tree or other vegetable.
This appears a quite uncalled for attempt to bring the
text into line with popular exoteric fables about re-birth
in all sorts of animal and vegetable forms.   Such a view,
however, quite ignores the clear implication of the text
that those who re-enter a womb do so according to their
Karma while those who go to the *Sthāṇu* do so according to their knowledge.   Accordingly we have translated it as the Fixed which is also its *primary* meaning.

The *Sthāṇu* is in fact the Fixed Pole of being,
Dhruva, the Pole Star, around which the Heavens turn,
the *Stauros* or Pillar that is referred to in Gnostic writings, the pillar of Wisdom that stands through all the
ages.   The Kabala also knows it, terming it the Middle
Pillar.   Primarily it is the Higher Self, the Thumb-
like *Purusha*.   He who, as a previous verse told us, alone
IS To-day and To-morrow.   It is the Pillar which mediates between Earth and Heaven, the Earth of the
physical universe and Heaven of the *Mahat* and, as
always, on account of its central position, it is the
Place of Power.

The Thumb-like *Purusha* is, however, we may remember, a triple Flame, for it is the triple Human Monad
sometimes   referred   to   as   *Ātma-Buddhi-Manas*.[1]   It
is not *Manas* alone that is the Fixed Pillar but *Manas*
as united to the two higher Flames and therefore the
Path of Knowledge or the Path of the Gods leads the
Soul right up to the Great World of the *Mahat* and is
so described in the Gita and in other Upanishads: "Fire-
light, Day, the Bright Fortnight, the six months of the
Sun's Northern Path, then going forth, the Brahma-
knowers go to *Brahman*."[2]

[1] See *Shwetāshwatara Upanishad*.
[2] *Gita* 8, 24.

In this description the stages on the Path are symbolised by Times, which, as Shankara truly says, are really Gods. On leaving the physical body the Soul finds itself in the red Fire-light of the Desire world. Knowing, however, its bright and flickering forms to be illusions which would bind it, it passes on to the steady Day-light of the higher *Manas*, that which shines steadily throughout the ages. Thence it unites with the waxing Moon of the *Buddhi*, passing at the Full into the Six Months of the north-going Sun, the Great World of the *Mahat*.

Certain Upanishads[1] add some further stages. From the six north-going Months the Soul passes into the Year or in other words masters the complete cycle of being. Thence to the Sun of the *Purusha* or *Shānta Ātman*, thence to the Moon of the *Mūla Prakṛiti*, thence to the Lightning of the Central Power. From this point a non-human being (*amānava purusha*) leads them to the *Brahman*, or, in other words, the Path passes beyond humanity altogether. "Of these there is no return." We need not, however, concern ourselves with these transcendent stages but will pass on to the description of the other Path, the Path of Karma, as given in the Gita:—

"Smoke, Night, the Dark Fortnight, the Six Months' of the South-going Sun, thence the yogi, having gained (only) the Moonlight, returns."[2]

In other words, the Soul that loses itself in the smoky vapours of desire reaches, not the Day of illumination, but the Night of ignorance. Thence he passes to the Waning Moon. Whereas, to the Soul with Knowledge, the Light gets clearer as it soars away from the body, to the ignorant, desire-bound Soul, everything gets

---

[1] e.g., *Chandogya Upanishad*, 5, 10.
[2] *Gita* 8, 25.

darker and darker for it feels that it is leaving the light of physical life, the only light it ever knew farther and farther behind it. Thence it passes to the Six Months of the south-going Sun. The deep and universal levels of its being are always there, however ignorant the Soul. Nevertheless, as a conscious entity, it does not perceive them. Beyond it seems only the blackness of the wintering year and it shrinks back, away from Reality and re-enters the delusive but familiar Moonlight, the Light that is reflected in the Moon of Matter. This is called obtaining the Moonlight. In it the Soul dreams pleasantly or unpleasantly, according to its previous deeds, until, the desire-energy stored in the psychic structures built up while in earth life becoming exhausted, the attractions of the ties left behind in the physical world make themselves felt and once more the Soul projects its ray into a suitable womb, and, in due course is born once more. As we read in the *Brihadāranyaka Upanishad*:

> "Being attached, the subtle mental self along with its *karma* goes to that to which it is attached.
> Coming to the end of the fruits of its deeds done in this world it returns from that world to this for (further) action.
> Thus the man who desires."[1]

These are the two paths of the Soul after death, the Path of Knowledge, leading to Release and the Path of Karma, leading to rebirth down here.

(8) *The Purusha who wakes in those that sleep, bodying forth desire after desire, That is indeed the Pure, That the Brahman, That the Deathless. In It are contained all the worlds and none ever goes beyond It. This verily is That.*

[1] *Brihadāranyaka Upanishad* 4, 4, 6.

(9) *As Fire, though one, having entered the world, becomes similar in form to every form (in which it burns), so the One Inner Ātman of all beings corresponds in form to every form (it ensouls) and yet is still outside them all.*

(10) *As Air, though one, having entered the world, becomes similar in form to every form (in which it dwells), so the One Inner Ātman of all beings corresponds in form to every form and yet is still outside them all.*

(11) *As the Sun, the Eye of the all beings, is not stained by the external defects of the eyes, so the One inner Atman of all beings is not stained by the misery of the world, being outside it.*

Having set forth the Paths of the Soul the Teacher takes up the other point, the nature of the Secret Eternal *Brahman*, which, from the human point of view, is the Secret Power which manifests in the Thumblike *Purusha* in the heart. That *Purusha*, as a constructed form is not of course as such the *Brahman*, but, on account of its central position, it is the point through which shines forth the Fiery Power which is the only aspect under which the ultimate unity of the *Parabrahman* can be known to us. Just as during the Night of *Pralaya* the ceaseless Breath of the Unbreathing One rests not, so in the little night of man the sleepless central Power remains awake and is the fount of energy which creates the desire-clothed images of dream.

Lest, however, we should be tempted to suppose that because it gives life to and ensouls the desire-images, it is therefore a power that belongs to the Ignorance, something to be transcended, the text hastens to add that it is the utterly Pure, the Deathless *Brahman* itself. It is the one ultimate and only Power. In itself it is neutral to all questions of high or low, good or evil. We have seen how it manifests on all the levels of the Cosmos and it is as indifferent to the forms it ensouls as is the Sun to the objects it shines upon. It vivifies the murderous phantasies of a maniac as readily as the compassionate aspirations of a saint, just as the power of electricity will slay a man or give him warmth and light indifferently. Like the Fire which is its symbol it is so pure that nothing can defile it. Arrange the conditions suitably and it will manifest, but whether its manifestation shall be a blessing or a curse depends on those conditions arranged by us. It is we and we alone that are responsible for the nature of its manifestation. We arranged the fuel and it is we who must abide the result. It is the Power which will "make of thee a God," the Power that sends the Soul soaring on wings of flame to Heaven; it is also the Power which makes of man a devil, vitalising his thoughts of lust and cruelty and thus hurling him to hell. Truly, a terrible Power, one that resembles not at all the loving heavenly Monotheos of popular religious phantasy, one from which men may well shrink back in fear, though, as the Teacher has told us, the wise and heroic do not.

Like fire, in itself unmanifest, but taking the form of whatever fuel it is invoked into, like air, itself formless, but taking the shape of the beings who breathe it, or, we may add, like light taking the form of the mirror which reflects it, so this one secret Power becomes shaped in accordance with the nature of the forms, which reflect it, the forms which it ensouls. And yet, just as with all these elemental Powers, the Fire is more than all the fires on earth, the Air more than all the breaths and the Light more than all its reflections, so is that Power more than all its manifestations.

"Having established this whole universe with one portion of My being, I remain."[1]

[1] *Gita* 10, 42.

It has also the utter neutrality of the Elemental
Powers.   Like Fire which will warm a man or burn down
his house with the same utter detachment from results,
like Water which will quench our thirst or drown us,
like the Sun itself which gazes with an equal eye upon
scenes of peaceful cultivation or of bloody massacre,
so does the one Power enter into and ensoul our thoughts
and feelings.   Whether those thoughts are good or evil,
as we count such, is our responsibility who framed
them, just as it is our responsibility if we use precious
books instead of coal for feeding our kitchen fires.   It
will send forth a life-boat's crew upon its errand of
mercy or it will hurl an army like a burning fire across a
continent.   The Sun is the source of the energy stored
in coal or oil but it cannot be held responsible for the
uses to which we put these substances.

The common taste for raising ultimate problems
before understanding the proximate ones will surely
object that if it is the one universal Power then the selection of the fuel, the framing of the thoughts, must also
be its work and its responsibility.   We can only
say that it is not so in any sense which can be rightly
applied to the term.   The independent centre of the
Ātman that shines in each of us has its own inalienable
creative freedom, which, *as long as it maintains its separateness*, can do or not do at what must be termed its own
will, on its own responsibility and reaping its own
fruits.   What happens when that separateness is dissolved is another matter and one to which terms like responsibility do not apply.   The source of all the evils
in the world is to be found in the sense of separateness,
the Ego.   Beyond the Ego there is and can be no evil.
Nothing has ever touched the stainless purity of the
'Above' and nothing ever will, any more than the defects of our eyes can ever effect the all-pervading vision
of the Sun.

Chapter V

The exhaustion of fuel leaves the Fire just what it always was, the shattering of the mirror leaves the Light untouched. Birth and death apply solely to the forms which come and go; That which gives life to them is Birthless and Deathless. These are but words, the sort of words, moreover, that we are in the habit of using in such contexts, having, too often, little more content than vague emotional aspiration. But words are of no use. Where shall we find the deep Reality to which they should apply, the Flaming Power itself "in which dwell all the worlds"? That Power is, as we have said, not the benevolent God of popular religion; neither is it the respectably abstract, 'philosophical' *Ātman* of ordinary current *Vedānta*. It is the cold black Flame that burns but is not hot, burning with an intensity not to be found in the heart of the hottest star, and yet not hot, for not even the most delicate petals of a flower are scorched by it. It is in all things or rather, as the Gita says, not It in them but they in It. It burns unquenched in the depths of the Waters but it burns equally in the treeless plains of Space. And it is burning all around us at this moment. Every form we see is but the smoke which veils its hidden Flame, all that we hear the echo of its throbbing soundless Sound. But where is the eye that shall see It? Where the ear that shall hear It? As another Upanishad says: "what eye shall see the Seer, what ear hear the Hearer?"

And yet It is there: we know that It is there. Words fail us utterly and are flung aside as useless. Even the mind turns back maddened by its inability to grasp this Wondrous Being. We claw the air and grasp at emptiness and all the time it is the Power that moves the clutching hands, That which sustains the circling flight of mind.

It is the ultimate Wonder, the 'secret and eternal Great One'; Fire which does not burn, Light which is not seen, Support which cannot be touched, Life which does not move.

"Unmoving the One is swifter than the mind,
The Gods attained It not for It had gone before.
Standing it passes others though they run.
It moves: It moves not: It is far: It is near.
It is within all this and It is outside all this."[1]

What shall we say of It save in the words of the *Kena*:—

"The eye goes not There, neither the speech nor mind,
We know not, we do not understand how one should teach It,
For it is other than all that is known and other also than what is unknown.
Thus we have heard from the ancient Seers who explained it to us."[2]

It is the ultimate, the Rootless Root of Being, "and none can ever go beyond it." This verily is That.

(12) *The One Controlling Power, He who makes his one form into many, is the Inner Ātman of all beings—the Wise who realise Him as standing in the self, to them and not to others belongs eternal bliss.*

(13) *Constant amidst (the forms) which come and go, (essential) Consciousness of all the conscious beings, the One amidst the Many, He who dispenses the objects of desire—the Wise who realise Him standing in the self, to them and not to others belongs eternal bliss.*

[1] *Ishopanishad* 4 and 5.
[2] *Kena Upanishad* 1, 3.

Chapter V

(14) This is That—thus they know—the supreme indescribable bliss. How, indeed, shall I understand It? Does it shine of itself or is it a reflection?

(15) Not There shines the Sun, nor Moon nor Stars nor these Lightnings, still less this (earthly) Fire. In His shining all (these) shine after Him. By His Light all this is illumined.

After watching our fruitless attempts to grasp that One Thing, the wonderful Controlling Power, in the world outside us, the Teacher repeats once more what he has so often told us, namely, that It is to be found within and not without. It may be and indeed is the Power which calls forth all forms, the Power which wields the heavenly bodies as a child would wield a stone in a sling, the One Power which ensouls the many forms it has created as the one Sun is reflected in a thousand pools of water. Nevertheless, although present there, it can never be grasped within those forms. No far-ranging explorations of the great or small without us, not all the keen probings of the all-dissecting mind, can ever reveal It to us if we have not first found It in the one spot where it is Self-luminous, the Point in the centre of our hearts.

It is true that what is above is also below and what is within is also without. Nevertheless we must remember that the two Poles of *Purusha* and *Prakriti* through which It manifests are the two Poles of Light and Darkness. It is no doubt present in the forms outside us but Its presence there is as the Root of the *Prakriti* and it is shrouded over by the latter's Darkness. It is there and can be felt there by that mode of massive feeling that belongs to the Darkness but such feeling is too universal and too hidden and instinctive for it to satisfy us as self-conscious beings. Therefore we are directed to the other Pole; we are to seek It rather as the Root of consciousness than as the Root of Form, though, indeed, It is both. We wish and need, not to unite our deep instinctive being to Its being—such union is there all the time—but to unite our *consciousness* to It, and thus to annul the sense of separateness that is the source of all our ills. Only in such union is there healing for the Soul.

We are to look within our hearts to find That which is constant amid the flux of thoughts, feelings and sensations, the psychic states that come and go incessantly like clouds that float in the sky. What is the inner Sky in which float all these psychic clouds, what that unchanging Blue in which they have their being? Whence comes that conscious Light that lights them all as they sweep through the heavens of the psyche? Each thought, each feeling, each sensation as it passes is lit up with the light of consciousness. Whose is that consciousness and from what mystic Fount within us does it stream forth?

This is the direction in which we must seek and this is the type of question we must ask if we would belong to that brotherhood of the Wise who realise His presence as within the self, they who enjoy eternal bliss, they and no others.

The Light-Stream flows outwards; we must go inwards if we would find its source. Like salmon in the breeding season we must ascend that River, recking nothing of obstacles; as an arrow we must shoot ourselves against the current to the Source from which it springs. There and there only shall we find the Bliss that throbs at the heart of being, the Bliss that is the World's Desire and whose reflections in the forms that come and go, lend the attractiveness to our desires.

When that Point is reached a wonderful sight is seen. The Waters of Light that we have traced back, narrowing and narrowing to their Source, are seen to widen out again on the other side into a great Ocean of calm and living Light whose blue waters shine with a radiance never before beheld.

> "Then felt I like some watcher of the skies
>   When a new planet swims into his ken;
> Or like stout Cortez, when with eagle eyes
>   He stared at the Pacific—and all his men
> Look'd at each other with a wild surmise
>   Silent, upon a peak in Darien."

Softly the waters rise and fall in ceaseless rhythm and with each wave a throb of bliss pulses through the watching Soul, so that, forgetting all, it longs to plunge for ever in their cool depths.

It is the eternal Summer Sea, the Sea whose waters wash for ever the inner shores of being. A channel leading to it is to be found in the heart of every living creature and all these separate channels lead to the same Sea, one and all-pervading, in whose Waters all sense of separateness is lost. Therefore we are bidden to seek the Way in our own hearts for only there shall we find it.

As it bursts upon our view we realise that it is That for which all our life we have been seeking. Nor has our search been confined to this one life alone. Spurred on by a dim memory of having known it long ago, we have wandered on and on through life after life in a darkness so great that we have almost forgotten that this Sea of Light existed. Always it has lured us on over the next range of hills and always when we got there the view disclosed has been of a country similar to the ones we have been wandering through so long. Only when we realise that the blue light that makes those far hills so magical comes from a Light that shines within our eyes do we call a halt to our endless wanderings, and, turning back upon ourselves, enter the Stream that leads us to the Sea.

Once there there can be no more disappointment, no more frustrated longings. The Sea! The Sea! There are those waters out of whose depths all life has risen: there is our Home. There is "the great Achilles whom we knew" and There, rising from the starry foam upon the surface stands Aphrodite Uranios, the *Heavenly* Aphrodite, she who "clothed round with the World's Desire as with raiment" has beckoned us throughout the ages from within the countless forms of our desires.

> "White rose of the rose white water,
> A silver splendour, a flame,
> Bent down into us that besought her,
> And earth grew sweet with her name."

This is it! This is it! Thus indeed cry out those who win to the Vision, those who bathe in the indescribable bliss of those Waters. They know that this is what they have sought so long but even they are at a loss to know how to understand that which now lies before them. This Light, for instance, this blue Radiance that lies upon the waters as the haze upon a summer's day. Whence does it come? Only gradually do they come to understand that it is the Light of lights, the ultimate radiance of Being. For in that Inner Sea there is no Day and Night, no Sun of life, no Moon of death, no Stars of separateness. The Lightnings of the mind are stilled in peace: the smoky fires of desire are extinguished.

There indeed is "the Light that never was on sea or land" for there is the essential Light by which shine all the elemental lights below, the one true Light without whose shining there could be no light at all.

"For there shall be no Night there; and they need

no candle, neither light of the Sun; for the Lord God giveth them Light: and they shall reign for ever and ever."[1]

[1] *Revelations* 22, 5

CHAPTER VI

(1) *With Root above and Branches below is this Primaeval Fig Tree. That is indeed the Pure, That the Brahman,
That is termed the Deathless. In It are contained all the
worlds and none ever goes beyond It. This verily is That.*

We are here introduced to the symbol of the Great
Tree, the Tree of Life whose leaves are for the healing
of the Nations,[1] one which was known to all the ancient peoples. The Scandinavians knew it as the
sacred ash-tree, Igdrasil, with its roots in the death-
kingdoms and its branches in the sky. In his poem to
Hertha, the Norse Nature-Goddess, Swinburne writes
of:—

> "The tree many rooted
> That swells to the sky
> With frondage red-fruited
> The life-tree am I;
> In the buds of your lives is the sap of my leaves:
> Ye shall live and not die."

The Egyptians worshipped the sacred sycamore
fig-tree, the Aztecs of Mexico had their sacred agave
plant and the ancient Sumerians of Eridu tell of a wondrous tree with "Its roots of white crystal stretched
towards the deep, its seat the central place of the earth,
its foliage the couch of the primeval Mother. In its
midst was Tammuz."[2] The following up of this sub-

---

[1] *Revelations* 22, 2.
[2] D'Alviella: *The Migration of Symbols*, p. 157.

246

ject would take us all over the world for the Tree is in fact a symbol of the Great World Mother, the Goddess of Nature who nourishes all life with the milk of her breasts. Hence the choice by the Egyptians of the syca-more fig with its milky juice and hence the fact that the three most sacred trees of the ancient Indo-Aryans were the *ashwattha*, the *bat* or *banyan* and the *udumbara*, all of them being species of fig tree.

The name *ashwattha* is usually derived from *a-shwa-stha*, "not standing till to-morrow," but, while this is an appropriate enough description of the world which is ever passing away before our eyes, there is an earlier account which goes deeper for it tells how Agni, the Fire, hid in this Tree for a year (the cycle of mani-festation) in the form of a Horse, no doubt the famous Stallion of which we have already written.[1] This sym-bolism is of great significance as it links up with the statement already quoted that Tammuz was in the midst of the Sumerian World Tree, and also, perhaps, with the growth of an erica tree round the coffin of the dead Osiris, for both these 'dying Gods' were symbols of the *Ātman*, the Secret Fire, dismembered and im-prisoned in the world.

There is, however, one peculiarity of the Indian

---

[1] *Taittirīya Brāhmaṇa.* III. viii, 12, 2. See Tilak's *Gita Rahasya* on Gita 15, 1. The same symbolism occurs in the *Mahābhārata Anushāsana Parva*, section 85. We may also note that one of the meanings of *ashwa* is 'seven,' that a vignette in the Egyptian *Book of the Dead* represents the sacred Sycamore Fig-Tree with seven branches, that the same is true of many representations of the Assyrian Tree of Life, and, finally, that the trunk of the famous many-breasted statue of Artemis of Ephesus is divided into seven levels, five of which are filled with representations of living creatures. See Mackenzie, *The Migration of Symbols*, pp. 162-169 for drawings of these. This note and most of what has just been written has been taken from my *Yoga of the Bhagavat Gita* where the same subject is treated.

tradition that is not, so far as I know, found else-where, namely, that the Root of the Tree is said to be above and the Branches beneath, whereas all the other World Trees have their Roots in the under-world and their Branches in the Sky. This tradition in India goes back to the Rigveda which speaks of *Varuṇa* "who sustaineth erect the Tree's stem in the baseless region. Its rays, whose root is high above, stream downward. Deep may they sink within us and be hidden."[1] The tree is, in fact, rooted in the unmani-fest Darkness of the Parabrahman, which is usually sym-bolised as 'above' though in fact it is no less truly 'be-neath' as well. From that transcendent rooting-place it sends down its trunk of manifestation through the worlds, and on that trunk are seven main branches each of which splits into countless branchlets and twigs. Nevertheless the Trunk itself is one for it is the Tree of the Mother, the great *Mūla-prakṛiti*, the Substance of the universe. The sap that runs in its veins is the very Life of all beings and on its branches hang the Stars themselves.

On all levels this Tree exists and therefore in man, the microcosm, we find it in the structure of the nervous system which resembles a tree, rooted in the brain and ramifying all over the body. This, however, is on the purely physiological level and concerns man's physical body alone. Of far more significance is the Tree of the human psyche, the Tree which has its roots 'above' in the pure consciousness of the *Ātman* and its branches in the thoughts, feelings and sensations of normal psychic life. Here again the Trunk is the Middle Pillar of *Manas*, that which stands connecting the ramifying network of Roots above with the similarly ramifying Branches beneath. To reach the Roots of our being,

---

[1] *Rig Veda*, I, 24, 7.

therefore, we have to leave the Branches that wave in the breeze of the outer world, those branches laden with the sticky sprouts of sensation, climb the unitary central Trunk and thus reach the Roots that dwell in the Ocean of Life.

This is the Tree, the Tree of the psyche, that is climbed by the *Rāja-yogi*. The other, the purely physiological one, which is, however, not without its interest on its proper level, may be left to the *Hatha yogi* with his stretchings and strainings, his *netis* and *dhoutis*, his *bandhas* and *mudras* etc., all designed to act upon the physical body in general and the nervous system in particular.

The text goes on to state that this Tree is indeed the *Brahman*, the Pure, the Deathless which none ever goes beyond. This statement will perhaps surprise those who make a rigid dualism of the *Purusha* and the *Prakriti*, regarding the latter as something evil, something to be transcended. Hence many interpreters have held that the latter part of the verse applies not to the Tree itself but to That in which it is rooted, or, at most, to the Root above. Such a view, however, seems uncalled for. The text has no such indications. We should remember the great Upanishadic teaching that "all *this* is verily the Brahman" and not attempt to make an ultimate dualism where only a relative one exists.

Admittedly the Tree is the great *Prakriti*; admittedly the *Prakriti* is the source of all matter and material objects and admittedly these objects are the source of bondage for us. Nevertheless the *Purusha* and the *Prakriti* are not independent realities but only the two Poles of one Reality. Neither could exist without the other and where there is one there are both. The Gita teaches that both are eternal and in truth the Motherhood of the *Prakriti* is no less Divine and no less Pure than the Fatherhood of the *Puruṣha*.

It is true that for purposes of yoga the *Puruṣha* is considered as in some sense higher than the *Prakṛiti* (see verse 7 of this chapter) but we should be careful lest we are ensnared in webs of our own weaving. All is the One Reality and in truth the Waters of the Great Sea are as Pure as is the Sky which is reflected in their depths. Everything depends upon the point of view from which it is seen.

There is an old manuscript recently reprinted which claims to have originated in the famous Brotherhood of the Rosy Cross.[1] One of its plates depicts the World Tree with the Three Worlds on its trunk. Six hands issue from them and seek to grasp the fruits of the Tree. Concerning them the text states "poor fools ......they grasp for pieces when they could obtain the whole. They seek for quiet and cannot find it."

A seventh hand grasps the trunk where the divided branches return to unity "but even this hand is still far from the roots of the tree, only holding and grasping the secret from the outside and cannot yet see it from the inside."

In the very centre of all the spheres is a single Eye, the Eye of Wisdom which alone can understand the tree.

"This Eye looks with the greatest peace upon the wonders of all movements and also looks through all the other eyes (scattered in the spheres), wandering about outside of the rest in the unrest, all those eyes which want to see for themselves without the right eye of Wisdom, from which they have received all their seeing power."

It is from the point of view of that Eye that the Tree is described as the utterly Pure. Truly no one

---

[1] *Secret Symbols of the Rosicrucians*; Engelke.

goes beyond it for beyond it is the Nothing.

(2) *Whatever there is, this whole Universe,[1] has come forth from and vibrates in* Prāṇa. *The Great Fear, the raised Thunderbolt—those who know that become Immortal.*

(3) *From fear of It Fire burns, from fear of it the Sun shines: from fear* Indra *and* Vayu[2] (*perform their functions*) *and Death advances as the fifth.*

The word *Prāṇa* here is not employed as one of the pair *prāṇa* and *apāna*, still less as one of the set of five, but should be taken in its most general sense of Life, the One Life that is in all beings. Out of that Life the whole universe has come forth and in it it moves in its constant vibratory rhythm. For Life is essentially movement or, rather, it is the motionless cause of movement in all things, an inbreath followed by an outbreath, life followed by death. In this general sense both life and death as opposed movements are included in Life; the inbreath or movement towards the pole of Spirit being life and the out-breath, the movement towards matter, death.

In all manifestations the opposites are for ever linked together and these two opposed movements are no exception. Death follows life and then again life follows death with the same inevitability as nights and days succeed one another. Of all that is manifested this ceaseless rhythm is the ruler and nowhere can there be anything which is exempt from the alternation of day and night. Hence, though all things are in Life and Life in all things, yet Life is not the same as life for the latter is linked indissolubly with death. All things dwell in eternal Life but if we seek that Life

1 *Jagat*, literally, the Moving-Thing.
2 Air.

we must do so in the Night no less than in the Day,
must learn to recognise it in the inturned stillness of what
we term death no less than in the exuberant outpouring
known by us as life.

This distinction between Life and life is one of
the utmost importance for if we fail to grasp it we shall
utterly fail to understand the teaching. As a child
makes castles out of sand only for them to be levelled
again by the inflowing tide, as a man creates a garden
out of a wilderness only for it to be reabsorbed by the
jungle when his watchfulness is removed, as the sun in
spring draws forth the plants from the dark bosom of
earth only for them to re-enter that earth in autumn, so
does the gaze of Spirit draw forth forms from the matrix
of the Great Mother only to have them reabsorbed in
Her when that gaze slackens as the Great Breath passes
into its opposite phase. The life of the forthcoming and
the death of the return are alike movements within the
one great Life. Both must be accepted if we seek the
Deathless State. Hence it is that for all manifested
beings, death hovers as the shadow of life. None can
escape it and therefore the Ruler, the ceaseless Breath
of Life is the great Fear, the thunderbolt upraised over
the heads of all that live. Always has death been termed
the great Leveller, the Sea which levels down again the
sand castles which life, like a child at play, builds up and
then abandons. With the laying of the first stone come
into play the forces that will ultimately level the house
once more to the ground as certainly as with the shooting
of an arrow are born the forces that will bring that arrow
back to earth. Therefore has it been said that from our
birth our death is also fixed, its mode and time can
be foreseen by those who read the heavens at that moment.

Thus do all things pass into their opposites. That
which is born shall die and that which dies shall be

reborn. "Fixed is death for the born and fixed is birth for the dead. Therefore thou shouldst not grieve over the Inevitable."[1]

But we do grieve and persist in grieving. The reason is not far to seek. We cling to the mode of life because it is the mode of self-assertion, the mode by which the ego rushes forth upon the universe to have and hold for itself. But all things must be paid for. Every gain is a loss; every getting has in its heart the seeds of an inevitable taking-away and every step we take forward raises the Thunderbolt of Doom higher above our heads. Deep in our hearts is the knowledge of this Law because deep in our hearts is the Fount of Life itself, Life which is life and death and knows their interchange, Life which is far beyond the personal outgoing which we know as life. Therefore it is that Fear dogs our footsteps and the death-hounds of the Moon pursue relentlessly our radiant Solar chariot. Did not guileful lunar Isis set a poisonous serpent in the path of solar Ra, the King of Gods ? Yet Isis is the Goddess of Wisdom and only pursues us in the form of the Fear because we will not worship her. "He who seeks his life shall lose it." It is because we cling so frantically to life alone that we are unable to see that death is also Life. That is the wisdom; the Wisdom that is the balance of the opposites. Out of the Marriage of the Sun and Moon is born the Stone of the Philosophers. "They who know That become Immortal."

But if we seek that Immortality we must seek the Life that is beyond life and death, beyond them because it is the unity of which they are the two poles. All who do not willingly yield themselves to its secret rhythm are ruled by its thunderbolt of fear. This applies not to men alone but to the whole creation, including the

[1] Gita 2, 27.

living Cosmic Powers that are the Gods, for though their Day may last through countless ages, it is followed by a Night of equal length.

> "Through *Prāṇa* the Gods live; so also do men and animals. *Prāṇa* is indeed the life of (all) beings. Therefore *Prāṇa* is known as the Universal life."[1]

Hence, as Cosmic Powers, manifested in the elemental Powers of this level, it is literally true that their activities are a running away from the raised Thunderbolt,·for all manifestation is a pulling out of the matrix, a process which creates a tension which is the essence of what we know as fear. Therefore, as we have said before, all beings, Gods and men alike, have to keep moving, running away from the pull towards their own Centre, if they are to remain manifested.

The verse has another meaning too for the Gods are also the presiding Powers of the various senses in man and it is no doubt with this fact in mind that the text mentions five. Here too there is the same running, the same press of activity, to avoid the pull to the Centre.

And yet that pull is quite inescapable. However far we may run, however vigorously we may assert ourselves, it will wear us down in the end. Slowly our strength fails and inevitably we yield to the pull and pass into our opposite. In so far as, in the attempt to live we have created a self that is far removed from the Central Self, to that extent we seem to lose all of our self in passing into the Night of death. Only those who can poise their being in the Centre, can gaze on all sides with an equal eye, can welcome Night as warmly as they welcome Day, can look, that is, on life and death as but the severed halves of Life, only they are free from the Fear that rules the world and only they are the Knowers of

[1] *Taittirīya Upanishad.*

Life, the winners of Immortality.

(4) *If one has been able to understand (It) here before the loosening of the body then indeed is one fit for embodiment in (all) the worlds of creation.*[1]

(5) *As in a mirror so is It seen in the self (of this physical plane); as in a dream so in the World of the Fathers; as in waters, so in the World of the* Gandharvas *and as Light-and-Shade, so in the* Brahma *World.*

The last verses set forth to us the Life that is at the heart of all creation, the Life of which life and death as we know them are both aspects. The present verse goes on to say that here and now, before the loosening of the physical body in death, this Life is to be realised. We have already referred to the fact that this is always the attitude of the true inner Teaching which never postpones anything till after death. Whatever can be realised at all can be realised here and now, for "that which is There is also here" and what is not here in some form or other is not anywhere at all. He who thinks, as do most of the exoterically religious, that he will be inducted into the mysteries of Being merely by the process of changing this state of existence for another is grievously mistaken. He who has not known the nature of Life and Immortality here will not know them simply by dying.

He, on the other hand who while here in the very midst of life can realise the other side of his being, the other movement which we know as death, can realise it as much a part of his real Being as is the life-

---

[1] I have translated this verse just as it stands neither changing *chedashakat* 'able' into *chennashakat* 'unable' as is hesitatingly suggested by Max Muller, nor with Shankara inserting so big an ellipsis as to change the meaning into its opposite, nor with Madhva reading *Swargeshu* instead of *sargeshu*.

movement, such a man has here and now mastered the cosmos. Poised in the Centre, nowhere is there any obstruction to his vision. He is made free of the entire universe; on all levels he can manifest in the manner appropriate to those levels, nowhere can there be any obstruction, any death for him. In a very real sense the whole universe with all its worlds, gross and subtle, has become his body. Others may dwell, or rather have to dwell, as guests within bodies. He alone is *worthy* of embodiment as he alone knows what a body really is and he alone is master of all bodies.

The perception of the great Life, however, varies in clarity according to the level of being on which it is seen. When seen within the ordinary waking self of this plane it is as a reflection in a mirror, something which can be seen but not grasped.

Above this level is the lunar world of the Fathers sometimes known as the astral world, the world of Desire. In that world the Life can be perceived more clearly for it manifests in a form comparable to the vivid figures that move about in our dreams. Moreover, on that level it is as the Desire-life that It manifests, and, as all know, desire is the very "stuff that dreams are made on," the force which sets their vivid life in motion.

Again, as in a mirror we see but the more or less static reflection of our own single face, so on this physical plane it is as a single form, one which reflects our outer appearance more or less closely, that the Life is seen. Such an image was known to the Egyptians as the *Ka* or double, sometimes known as the etheric double. Paracelsus says of it: "the whole of the Microcosm is potentially contained in the *Liquor Vitae* (the Life Fluid) ......in which is contained the nature, quality, character and essence of beings and which etheric Life-fluid in man may be looked upon as an invisible or hidden man—

so to say, his ethereal counterpart or reflection."[1]   This is the form which may sometimes be seen hovering near the fresh grave awaiting the complete decay of the body before itself disintegrating.[2]

As contrasted with this quasi-physical or 'etheric' image, which, as we have said, is relatively fixed in form, we find that in the Lunar Desire-world the Life is much more protean in its form, changing in appearance from moment to moment as do the shifting images of dream which are indeed its embodiments. The dream figures, though they seem external to ourselves, are in reality detached portions of ourselves, created by and ensouled by our Desire-life. It is on this plane that exist the images of our 'Fathers,' a fact of which psychologists have recently become aware and which they characteristically proclaim as a new discovery, though for ages it has been known to Eastern seers as the World of the Fathers.

Moving still higher up the Ladder of being we come to the Solar world of the *Gandharvas*.[3]   The *Gandharvas* of Vedik times were not the mere heavenly musicians that they became in Paurāṇik times any more than the Vedik *Varuṇa* was the mere God of pools and streams that he became later. Originally the *Gandharva* was a most mysterious heavenly being, "a measurer of space," who stands "erect upon the vault of Heaven." He is connected with the Sun and also with the Soma in its solar aspect.

---

[1] Paracelsus *De Generatio Hominis*: quoted in Hartmann's *Life of Paracelsus*.

[2] Egyptian funerary ritual and the practice of mummification seem, at least in part, to have been a process designed to preserve the *Ka* from such dissolution.

[3] The enumeration of these worlds is not always made in the same order. *Brihadāraṇyaka Upanishad* 4. 3. 33. clearly states that "a hundred fold the bliss of those who have won to the world of the Fathers is one bliss in the Gandharva world."

"High to heaven's vault hath the *Gandharva* risen,
  beholding all his varied forms and figures.
His ray hath gone abroad with gleaming splendour:
  pure he hath lighted both the worlds, the
                                        Parents."[1]

And again:

"Erect, to Heaven hath the *Gandharva* mounted,
  pointing at us his many coloured weapons;
Clad in sweet raiment, beautiful to look on, for
                                        he,
  as light, produceth forms to please us.
When as a Spark he cometh near the ocean, still
  looking with a vulture's eye to Heaven.
His lustre joining, in its own bright splendour,
  maketh dear glories in the lowest region."[2]

Quite clearly we are moving here in realms quite
different from those inhabited by the charming if somewhat lustful celestial musicians of later times. Truly
did Heracleitus teach that all things flow. Even the
Gods (or at least their Names) are bound upon the
turning Wheel of Fate and of them as of mortals it is
true that:

"Who ruled a King may wander earth in rags
  For things done and undone."

The *Gandharva* is in fact the higher Self, and the
world of the *Gandharvas* the plane of the higher *Manas*.
Hence the Solar symbolism and also the connection with
the higher aspect of the Soma, the sacred Drops of immortality. Hence also, as reflectors of the Harmony
of the *Buddhi*, the later view of them as heavenly musi-

[1] *Rig Veda* X; 85, 12 (Griffiths).
[2] Ibid X; 12, and 7 and 8.

cians. The original meaning persisted to some extent
in philosophy, for the term *Gandharva* is there used for
"the soul after death and previous to rebirth."[1] The
term corresponds in fact to the Daemon or Genius of
Greek and Roman thought, the Being who presided
over the birth of each man and protected him from
dangers if worthy of protection. Such a Genius was
also the source of inspiration, whence our modern use
of the term.

If, then, we ascend from the Lunar World of the
Fathers to the Solar world of the *Gandharvas* or Higher
Selves, we find the manifestations of the one Life becoming clearer still. It loses now its protean, ever-changing
characteristics and takes on a definite being which can
be perceived as having the same quality as the body of a
man seen within the clear green waters of a mountain
lake. The outline may wave and flicker with the movement of unseen currents but there can be no doubt as
to the definite identity of the form, to which indeed the
transparent waters impart a certain crystalline glamour
making the man appear a dweller of another world.

Just such are the characteristics of the Life as manifest in the high mental world of the *Gandharvas*. Gone
is the flame-like changeability, the emotional warmth,
the dreamlike and exciting personal intimacy of the
world of the Fathers. In this higher world all is bathed
in an emerald radiance, an impersonal crystalline brightness, a thrice-distilled clarity of cool and magic Light,
which will be recognised by one who sees it as similar
in character to the magical beauty of objects seen in the
water of a rocky pool.

---

[1] *Apte's Dictionary*. The necessity of the presence of a *Gandharva* (Pali *Gandhabba*) in addition to mere sexual union if a birth
was to take place was a matter of controversy among the Buddhist schools. See *Majjhima Nikāya* and *Abhidharma Kosha*.

The Yoga of the Kathopanishad

"Just, O King, as if in a mountain fastness there
were a pool of water, clear, translucent, and serene;
and a man, standing on the bank and with eyes to see,
should perceive the oysters and the shells, the gravel and
the pebbles and the shoals of fish as they move about
or lie within it[1]"—just so, indeed, is the one Life seen
in the clear waters of the Mānas Lake.

If we soar higher still to the great Brahma World
of the *Mahat*, the vision changes once more. The
symbolism becomes cosmic in character and we see the
Life as the eternal rhythm of Day and Night, the great
Northgoing and Southgoing movements of the Sun,
the cycle of the Seasons sweeping in slow deliberate
majesty around the starry Wheel of Fate during the
26,000 years of the great Precessional Year, the "Day
of *Brahmā* a thousand ages in duration" and the Night
of equal length, knowers of which, as the Gita tells us,
are the true Knowers of Day and Night.

We remember the Light and Shade of Chapter 3,
the Two (*Mahat* and *Buddhi*) who dwell in the upper
sphere of being, the Two who are reflections of the ultimate Two, the Father and the Mother from whose union
springs the *Brahma* World. All things down here have
their Shadows, phenomena that are trite enough to the
moderns who are so certain that they know all about
them, but which were of great significance to the
ancients.[2] All things not only have their Shadows but,
in the end, they pass into those Shadows which is why
the spirits of dead men are known as Shades. Light and
Shade. These two create the world. Is not the very

[1] *Dialogues of the Buddha*, I, page 93. Sutta on the Fruits of
the Life of a Recluse.
[2] We learn a little verbiage about light travelling in straight
lines and forthwith consider that we know all about shadows.
The ancient idea that a man could be bewitched through his
Shadow strikes us as quite absurd. Nevertheless it is true.

visual scene before us a play of Light and Shade upon the seven divine elemental colours? That and only that.

In this world all things are separate from their Shadows. A man is separate from the Shadow at his heels and life is separate from the death which dogs it. This is the very essence of manifestation, the making of two out of what is essentially one. The great Brahma World is also a manifested world and therefore there too are Light and Shade. But, compared to the worlds of plurality down here, it is a world of unity and in it the opposites are fused together in a wonderful embrace, a unity of two aspects, a pair which is yet one being. There life and death unite in Life which yet has its two movements. There, as Plotinus states, each being is itself and all the rest; in particular, each is itself and also its opposite. There are the two great Gods, *Mittra* and *Varuṇa*, Lords of the Day and Night. "Those who by Order (*rita*) uphold the Cosmic Order. Lords of the Shining Light of Order, *Mitra* I call and *Varuṇa*."[1] Sometimes the entire Lordship is considered as vested in *Varuṇa* alone and then it is He who dwells "at the River's Source surrounded by his Sisters Seven," He who supports the worlds of life, He in whom all wisdom centres as the nave is set within the wheel. He is "an Ocean far removed," one who wraps these regions as a robe, one who firm seated "rules the Seven as King," "who measured out the Ancient Seat, who pillared both the worlds apart as the Unborn supported Heaven." Lastly it is He who "O'erspread the Dark Ones with a Veil of Light," a clear reference to the marvellous union of Light and Shade that characterises the Brahma World, the Sacred Marriage in which the two are still two and yet their Son is One, the Son who is the Parent of his

[1] *Rig Veda* I. 23, 5.

Parents.[1] Such is the graded vision of the One Life
as it manifests in the many worlds of becoming, a vision
which culminates in that of Light-and-Shade, the
wonderful unity which we can only term Bright-Dark-
ness or Dark-Light, the union of the two opposing
movements, the Equilibrium which is the Throne of
Yoga.[2]

(6) *The wise, having understood the separate nature of
the senses, their rising and setting as of things that come into
being quite separate from himself, grieves not.*

(7) *Higher than the senses is the* manas. *Above the*
manas *is the Spirit.* (sattva, i.e., Buddhi). *Beyond the
Spirit is the Great Self* (Mahān Ātma): *above the great
Self is the Unmanifest.*

(8) *Higher than the Unmanifest is the* Purusha, *all-
pervading and devoid of any characteristic mark, which having
known, every living being is liberated and goes to the Deathless
State.*

Having described the modes in which the One Life
is present on all the levels of the universe and having
given us the signs by which we may recognise the vision
when we gain it, the Teacher goes on to recapitulate
the Path[3] which the ascent from one level to the other
may be made. As before we begin with the sense-

[1] *Rig Veda* VIII. 41. To avoid misunderstanding it should
perhaps be mentioned that the name *Varuṇa* as that of the Lord of
that World belongs to an older symbolism than does the name
Brahmā. With the rise of the latter into prominence *Varuṇa*
became a mere God of Waters.

[2] The Sanskrit term *Chhāyātapayoḥ* is a dual not a plural
term and its unity can only be rendered in English with the use
of hyphens. Incidentally it should really be Shade-and-Light
which, however, sounds clumsy.

[3] Chapter II verses 10 and 11.

life, the mire in which the foot of the Ladder is planted and which must be washed off in the Waters of Renunciation before the disciple can climb to the higher rungs. "Woe unto him who dares pollute one rung with miry feet. The foul and viscous mud will dry, become tenacious, then glue his feet to the spot, and, like a bird caught in the wily fowler's lime, he will be stayed from further progress."[1]

Therefore the first instruction is that we should study the nature of sensations as they rise and set within the heavens of the heart. "Learn from sensation and observe it, because only so can you commence the science of self-knowledge, and plant your foot on the first step of the ladder."[2]

We must observe carefully the nature of the sense life, not with any foolish idea that we can dispense with it altogether, but in order that we may gain that understanding of its laws that is the prelude to bringing it under complete control. Ordinarily we do not and cannot see our sense-life because we have identified ourselves with it. It is part of us and can no more be clearly seen by us than can our own bodies. Just as we need a mirror in which to see our own faces, so must we take the help of the Mirror of the Mind if we are to see and study the nature of the sense life. Only when we can stand back and see it as something separate from ourselves can we see it as it really is. Established in the mental being, we must observe the coming and going of sensations as we would observe the coming and going of insect life in our houses, noting carefully its various sorts, which sort is useful and which harmful, which is attracted by what and by what

---

[1] *Voice of the Silence.* Note the Gita's teaching that renunciation means renunciation of *attachment.*

[2] *Light on the Path.*

repelled. Then indeed we are on the high road to control, and, ceasing to identify ourselves with our sensations, cease to grieve as they come and go.

Above the senses is the mind (*Manas*), the central earth round which revolve the inverted heavens of sense, the 'I' which has now learned to hold itself separate and unattached. What is the nature of that *Manas*? Here again the Yogi must learn to centre himself in its very heart and to observe with care all that takes place around himself. He will see that within the heavens of sense revolves another heaven, the mental heaven of thought of which the stars are the separate thoughts that rise and set within him. One of the first things he will learn is that there is no disorder in that inner cosmos. The thoughts do not come and go at their own will nor is he himself the Ruler who controls their rising and setting. Patiently he sets himself to discover the laws of their coming and going and in this way detaches himself from them. Here, as in the outer world, only the wise man rules his stars, the fool is ruled by them. Another thing he will learn is that a star does not cease to be when it sinks below the western horizon and becomes invisible to him. Our thoughts do not cease to be or even cease to affect us simply because we cease to think them. They have indeed sunk below the rim of the world but only to circle round beneath us and the same evil thought that tormented and overcame me today, whose setting I watched with so much relief, will surely rise again tomorrow to continue its malefic work until I can learn to understand its true nature, and, by understanding, master it. In the microcosm of our hearts, as in the world, history repeats itself and moods return until we have learnt to control them by realising their separateness from our true Self. As above, so below; the starry Heavens are our greatest Teacher. He who has contemplated them with any understanding of their

eternal rhythms will not make the common mistake of
thinking that he has escaped from evil thoughts simply
because he has put them behind him nor that by hiding
his head under the blankets of hard work or outer activity
he will be able to free himself from the afflicting power
that he himself has bestowed upon his stars. The
thought to which we have once given life, ensouled
by that life, lives on perpetually, seen or unseen by us, a
blessing or a curse. Even in the death of the body
there is no death for it, and the thought "that rises
with us, our life's star, hath had elsewhere its setting."
Only in the recalling of the projected life, in the withdrawal of our Centre to a more inward level of our
being, is there mastery, freedom and peace, for only in
such withdrawal are we able to separate ourselves
from our thoughts and calmly contemplate the silent
revolutions of their heavens. Such withdrawal is
termed rising from the *Manas* to the *Sattva*, the level of
the Spirit, the luminous and harmonious *Buddhi*.[1]

The special difficulties of the ascent to the *Buddhi*
have already been described[2] and need not be repeated
again. The yogi has to pass right through himself, as
Hermes expresses it, "into a Body that can never die."
Plunging into the central Well of his heart he must go
through it to that inner Sea of which we have already
spoken. He must learn to place his being in that which
is beyond himself, in the divine and harmonious universe
of the *Buddhi* whence he will be able to master and
control all that is below. The Stars of that inner

[1] The term *sattva* has many meanings, such as true spiritual
essence, wisdom, purity, goodness and consciousness. It is also
the highest of the three *gunas*, the one which manifests light and
harmony. In the Gita, Arjuna is urged to rise above the opposites and stand firm in the *sattva*. It corresponds here, as
stated by Shankara, to the *Buddhi*.

[2] Chapter 3, verse 13.

Heaven are the guide and Teacher whose Voice alone he has heard before but whom he now sees face to face, with whom, indeed, he has become one.

Thence he ascends to the Great *Ātman* or Brahma World, the farthest bound of the manifested universe. Beyond again is the dark Matrix of the Unmanifest, the Mother of the worlds, and, at least in some sense, 'beyond' again is the calm all-seeing Light of the *Purusha* or *Shānta Ātman*, which pervades all the worlds, holding them in being with its contemplative gaze.

Like the light of the sky, that Light rests calmly on all that is but to nothing whatsoever is it attached or partial. Like the sky, too, it is devoid of any characteristic sign or mark by which it could be indicated.

(9) *Not within the field of vision stands Its form, nor with the eye can any see It. By the Heart, by the thought, by the mind is it framed. They who know That become Immortal.*

Its form or total being can never be within the field of perception for it is that which encloses all within its embrace. As Sri Krishna says, "having pervaded all this universe with one portion of my being, I myself remain."[1] Nor, indeed, can it be seen by the eye for it is "That which sees through the eye but which the eye cannot see."[2] The Objects which it illuminates can be seen but not Itself. Forever it is the Seer in all seeing, the Knower in all acts of knowledge. "Thou thyself alone knowest Thyself, O highest *Purusha*, Bringer-forth of beings, Lord of beings, Light of the Powers of Light, Lord of the world."[3]

[1] Gita 10, 42.
[2] Compare the words of Hermes: "it cannot be seen by the compounded element by which thou seest."
[3] Gita 10, 15.

Chapter VI

Nothing that is not itself the Light can know the Light. Only the *Purusha* who is in ourselves can know Itself. Whatever we can point out is but the framework in which that Light is shining. The sky is but the space between the branches of a tree, between the stars, or, at most, between two horizons. So too this Light is "framed by the Heart (*Buddhi*) by the thought, by the mind." All we can say of it is that it is That which lights up and fills all such frames, the Heaven in which float Sun and Moon and all the Stars. It is, as Hermes says, "That which is never tempted, which cannot be defined; that which has no colour nor any figure, which is not turned, which has no garment, which gives Light; That which is comprehensible unto Itself alone, which suffers no change, which no body can contain." And again: "That which is upward borne like Fire, yet is borne down like Earth, That which is moist like Water, yet blows like Air, how shalt thou perceive This with sense— the That which is not solid nor yet moist, which naught can bind or loose, of which in power and energy alone can man have any notion and even then it wants a man who can perceive the Way of Birth in God."[1]

No form that we ever give it can be its own form but merely some frame-work of mind, some constellation of the *Buddhi* within which its presence can be felt rather than seen. In itself it is beyond all such frame-works, the utterly unlimited, the endless Being of Light. For this reason it has sometimes been likened to Space, and the Buddhists as well as some Upanishads termed it the Void. They who know It have achieved the Deathless State, but only Itself can know itself and they who know it are those who have dissolved their separate being and become That which it is, the Source of all being whatsoever. They are those who have 'gone

[1] Hermetic Corpus, 13, 5.

beyond' by 'the Great Passing On,' those about whom
Nachiketas questioned the Teacher, saying that some
affirmed their existence, some their non-existence. In
the light of what has been written it can be seen that the
question is one which admits of no verbal answer. Such
a one has become the Light Itself, the very Root of Life,
it would be absurd to say of him that he has ceased to
be. On the other hand, being that Light, he has no
distinguishing marks, nothing of which or by which one
could point him out and say this is him, there, in such
and such a form he exists. In the Buddha's words:
"Vast, immeasurable and unfathomable like the mighty
ocean is the being of him who has won to the Truth.
To say that he exists does not fit the case and neither
does it to say that he exists no more." That which
exists (or rather that which Is) must be realised by each
for himself by treading the Path that the Teacher has
described. Once realised, all doubts are set at rest,
the Deathless State is reached.

(10) *When the five means of (sense) knowledge sink to
rest*[1] *together with the mind and the* Buddhi *also acts separately no more,*[2] *that is described as the Highest Path.*

(11) *This they understand as Yoga, the steady holding
fast of the senses. Then one is no longer drawn outwards.*[3]

[1] Literally 'stand down.'

[2] *vi-cheshtate; cheshtate* to act; *vi* separately, disjunctively.

[3] *Apramatta.* This is the opposite of *pramāda,* literally, care-
lessness, lack of vigilance, but a technical term in yoga which
is defined in Vyasa's commentary on *Yoga Sutras* 1, 30, as 'want of
development of the means of *samādhi.*' One who is *apramatta*
is thus one who is 'undistracted' as the word is translated by
Hume but in a rather special sense. He is no longer distracted
or drawn away from his central being by the sense objects which
for most men draw forth the psychic energy in a constant outward
stream.

Chapter VI

Yoga is the (knowledge of) arising and passing away.[1]

The instructions given in these verses find their parallel in the teachings of Hermes. "Withdraw into thyself and it will come; *will*, and it comes to pass; throw out of work the body's senses, and thy Divinity shall come to birth; purge from thyself the brutish torments —things of matter."[2] We must be careful, however, not to misunderstand the term 'will' as used in this passage. It does not refer to a stopping of the sense activities by any violent act of will as we understand it usually, that is, by any sort of grim setting of the mental teeth. Rather it refers to an entire concentration of the whole being on the attainment of the yoga which is indeed only attainable by him who cares for it more than for anything else in this or any other world. It cannot be attained by any sort of half-hearted efforts conducted in the 'experimental' spirit or out of mere desire for strange experiences. He to whom the yoga does not mean more than all else, he who is not ready if necessary to sacrifice everything else in order to attain it, had far better leave it alone altogether, and, if he is religiously minded, confine himself to the domain of ordinary exoteric religion, for to him yoga will be nothing but a source of sorrow and disillusion. By a whole heart it must be sought or it will be found to be mere vanity and vexation of spirit.

The five sense knowledges have indeed to stand down or sink to rest. They must, as Hermes says, be 'thrown out of work' in much the same way as the driving cogs of a motor are thrown out of work by opening

[1] See the similar use of the term in *Māṇḍūkya* 6 in connection with the state of *Sushupti*.
[2] *Hermetic Corpus* 13, 7.

the clutch which transmits the power to them. As long as that power is being transmitted, it is quite beyond our strength to hold the car still by clutching at the wheels. Just so it is quite impossible to still the senses by any setting of the teeth as long as power is being transmitted to them from the heart, the source of all power. As in the car, power is transmitted by what is quite literally a 'clutch'; that clutch must be opened, broken or released and then the wheels of the senses will in a short time sink to rest of themselves. A common notion, especially in the West, is that the yogi stills his senses by entering a hypnotic trance and that for this purpose he practises certain tricks with his eyes etc., in order to induce auto-hypnosis. Admittedly in such a trance the senses are stilled as long as the trance lasts, just as they are stilled every night when we enter the state of dreamless sleep. But such stilling is only temporary and when the would-be yogi emerges from his trance his senses awake once more in precisely the same condition as before trance supervened. Mere trance accomplishes nothing.

Neither is it in any way possible to hold the senses firm by mere strength: as soon expect to grip the flame of a lamp by a pair of pliers : what the Gita calls the axe of detachment is the only means by which any real stilling can be brought about.

The sixth chapter of the Gita describes certain details of seat, posture etc., that are useful for bringing about a preliminary state of relative calm. The actual details are the traditional ones which are suited to Indian bodies and an Indian environment. Others must modify them to their own needs, the essentials being a quiet place where there is no fear of being disturbed, a posture which is comfortable and steady but at the same time alert, and a breathing which is calm, light and steady.[1] The Upanishad makes no mention of these details which would have been generally known to its hearers and which in any case are only the preliminary clearing of the work-table before starting the real operations. They can do no more than provide favourable conditions in which to work. Even before them, the traditional instructions lay down two practices known as *yama* and *niyama* which may be loosely described as a control of the outer life and behaviour by a withdrawal as far as possible from disturbing pursuits and a practice of the ordinary methods of what is commonly known as self-control, the ordinary virtues which, as Light on the Path puts it, "create a fair atmosphere and a happy future" but which are "useless if they stand alone."

Incidentally it may be stated that there is a difference between the yogi and what is commonly known as the saint. He who is in favour of 'virtues' at all cost, and who seeks to attain a sort of hundred per cent virtuosity, is asking for trouble and will surely get it before he has gone very far. Above all things yoga is balance.

To return, however; when a preliminary, and, as it were, outer calm has been established it is necessary to proceed further and set about releasing the mental 'clutch.' This is done by standing back from the sensa-

[1] Yoga is the famous Middle Path and therefore we need a bodily poise which is neither associated in our minds with physical or discursive mental activity, nor, as for instance a lying-down posture, with going to sleep. Hence for those who can use it, the ideal nature of the cross-legged Lotus Seat. It offers a comfortable and steady posture with the body easily balanced and the spine erect, an important point this, for any bodily 'slouch' tends to destroy the necessary alertness of spirit. It also, by gathering the limbs, naturally favours an in-gathered state of the psyche. Nevertheless, if it cannot easily be maintained, if it causes pain in the knees, it is worse than useless and some other, more suitable to the individual, must be made use of.

tions as they come and go in their ceaseless stream, standing back so as to be able to watch them calmly as one would watch the traffic passing one's window. The self-identification with them, the sense of being personally involved in their comings and goings, must be broken and this can be achieved by identifying oneself with that which sees them instead of, as before, with what is seen; in this way even a painful sensation can be seen with the detachment of a surgeon operating on the body of a horribly mutilated victim of an accident. How can this be done? The only answer is 'by doing it.' We can all do it if we want to badly enough for, as (I think) the Buddhist *Abhidharma* literature has pointed out, there is an element of detachment present in all consciousness. We have only to cultivate it and the difficulties which loom so large in our path arise through the fact that we only very partially *want* to be detached, while much of us feels that such a state is altogether too 'dull.'

In any case detachment from sensations is only the first step. Those which follow are harder still. Besides the outer sensations there are the forms seen by the inner senses, the forms of memory, imagination and of phantasy in general and from all these which are 'things seen' the watchful, seeing Light of consciousness must be detached. Then there are feelings, all reducible to positive or negative forms of desire, the very life-blood of the senses, outer and inner. They too must be clearly seen as something quite apart from the seeing Light which can then be withdrawn from them so that the sensations themselves crumble into dust or at least stand like last year's plants, withered and brittle. "And then the heart will bleed, and the whole life of the man seem to be utterly dissolved." But the ordeal must be endured for the death of the body is the life of the soul, and, as Heracleitus wrote: we are "Immortal mortals, mortal Immortals, the one living the death and dying the life of the other."

Nor should any think that this killing out of the desire life is a path leading to a stone-like state of indifference, an icy loveless waste or even a 'tepid-death' such as is phantasied about by modern scientists as being the ultimate state of the universe. It is only the poisonous outflows, the *āsravas* as the Buddhists term them, that are thus to be cut off "like a palmyra tree." Our heart's blood flows away from a hundred gaping wounds in the skin of our psychic integrity and we are such fools that we mistake its deadly flow for living circulation, its clotting pools, fit only for ghouls and larvae, for the healthy life-essence. We must close the wounds and cut off the outer flow before we can regain our health, but that does not mean that no blood will flow within the veins of the healthy man. "The Soul of Things is sweet" and it is not from any icy waste that the Buddhas and other Great Teachers have come with their message of love and compassion.

When we have learnt to detach ourselves from the fluid, shape-changing forms of the lunar world we find ourselves in the clearer planetary world of thought, "these thoughts that wander through eternity". There again, we cannot still the movements nor fix the ever-changing patterns with the pliers of will. We must detach ourselves again and in detachment seek to understand their erratic movements for only then can we hope to bring them into control. Only when we have seen whence comes the power that sustains their circling flight can we once more open the clutch and let them sink to rest.

Beyond them is the sphere of the Fixed Stars, the calmly luminous world of the *Buddhi*. Here too there is movement, since, as long as we remain rooted in our personal selves, that sphere as a whole appears to rise

and set. Here is the hardest task of all, to pass beyond
ourselves so that that Sphere is seen no longer as a perpetual rise and set, focussed on a given point, but as it is
in itself, calm and at rest, an all-embracing living Sphere
of interlinked lights. This is what is meant by the
text's statement that the *Buddhi* also acts separately no
more. It no longer rises and sets, that is, it no longer
impinges upon individual action as the compensating,
ever-turning Wheel of Fate but shines in the constancy
of its own Divine Harmony. It may be added that in
practice this rise and set of the *Buddhi* results in the separate judgments which assert 'this is so-and-so,' 'that is
such-and-such,' the judgments that definitively establish
separate things and which are all that is known of the
Buddhi by scholastic philosophy. For the yogi these
judgments cease, for to him, as Plotinus also taught,
each is all and all is in each.

This, then, is the Yoga; the lowest rung is the 'steady
holding fast of the senses, the highest the calm mastery
of the Wheel of Fate.' But it is not a yoga to be practised
only in the hours of seated meditation. A quiet,
artificially arranged period for special effort is as useful
to the beginner as is a quiet, secluded space for him who
would learn to ride a bicycle. But the aim of the cyclist
is to be able to ride in safety in the busiest traffic and
the aim of the yogi is similarly not to enjoy himself in a
private peace of his own but to master his psycho-physi-
cal vehicles so that he can ride them serenely in the
midst of the roar and bustle of life.

In the last sentence of verse eleven the conclusion
of the whole matter is stated once more; Yoga is the
knowledge of arising and passing away, of the laws
which govern the rise and set of the manifold contents of the psyche, and, what is the same thing, of those
of the so-called external world. Once more we see
how all true yoga is one in all the separate traditions,

for this knowledge of arising and passing away is precisely that Conditioned Origination (*pratītya samutpāda*) that was what flashed upon the Buddha on the Fullmoon night of Enlightenment, the final insight into the causes of all things. He who knows how thoughts arise within the mind knows also how to bring about their cessation and what is true of thoughts is true of all things in the universe:

"By the stilling of the circling of the mind, all things within the universe are brought to rest."[1]

From another point of view also the yoga may be said to be, not merely the knowledge of, but itself the arising and passing away of all things. Yoga means union, and, just as it was by union with the Outwardness that all things came into being[2], so is it by union with the Inwardness that all things sink to rest. As for the nature of that Ultimate Reality in which all have their final abode, the ultimate Goal of the Yoga, it cannot be grasped by any of the partial manifestations that make up our psyche. How could it be? They are the parts and it is the Whole from which they took their rise. Therefore we read:—

(12) *Not by speech, nor by the mind nor by the eyes can It be compassed. How could It be comprehended other than by saying 'It is.'*

Speech is the activity which isolates and picks out particular individual forms while that Reality is, as another Upanishad puts it, *neti neti*, not this, not this. Mind is the activity which relates such individual forms

[1] Nāgārjuna's *Mahāyāna Vimshaka.* "*Sarve dharmā nirudhyante citta cakra nirodhataḥ.*"
[2] *Shwetāshwatara Upanishad* 6, 3.

in various patterns. How shall it deal with that which is beyond all relations. The eyes, and of course the other senses, even the inner ones which are intended to be included, reveal only a small portion of the lowest levels of cosmic differentiation; how shall they deal with the Whole out of which all these differentiations have taken place? Only in the deepest core of the heart is there found a certain profound knowledge which, itself beyond all words, can be rendered by the one word *asti*, 'It is.' Other schools, the Buddhists for instance, as well as some Upanishads, have held that even this expression goes too far since all existence means a standing forth and so a particular manifestation. They have therefore termed It the Shūnya, the Void, because It is nothing of all that we term things. This type of expression is also found in the Rig Veda for, we read that sages who searched within the heart "discovered the existent's kinship with the Non-existent."[1] Here the Non-existent (*asat*) is That which does not stand-forth, which is not manifest and is in fact identical with the 'It is' of our text. This becomes clear in the next verse which affirms:—

(13) *As 'is' It should be realised and also in reality as being both (is and is not).*
To him who realises It as 'is,' It's Real Being shines forth.[2]

In other words the utter incomprehensibility of

[1] *Rig Veda* X, 129, 4.
[2] The first half of this verse is difficult to translate but the general sense is clear. Seshacharri, following Shankara, renders it:—"He should be known to exist and also as he really is," while Hume translates: "He can indeed be comprehended by the thought 'He is' and by (admitting) the real nature of both (his comprehensibility and his incomprehensibility)."

Chapter VI

Ultimate Being (Be-ness has also been suggested, for neither 'Being' nor 'Real', i.e., thing-like, are satisfactory) is best approached by the positive or 'existent' approach. Otherwise there is risk of falling into the mere nihilism of which *Shūnyavāda* Buddhism was always being falsely accused and into which in fact some *Shūnyavādis* perhaps fell. Nevertheless, the movement of realisation, having grasped the fundamental is-ness of the Ultimate and having made its affirmation, must proceed further to the opposite negation, and then, with one foot as it were on each, must leap boldly into the arms of the utter Inexpressibility beyond. Beyond *Purusha* and *Prakriti*, (is and is not) he soars to ultimate *Brahman*; beyond Day and Night he gains the Sun-beyond-the-Darkness; beyond One and Many he attains the ultimate and magic Zero that is All. But why strain for words when we know in advance that they must and will betray us? Here more than ever are they but fingers pointing to the moon, "Whereof one cannot speak, thereof one must be silent."[1]

(14) *When all the desires that cling to the heart are detached, then the immortal becomes the Deathless. Here and now he attains the* Brahman.

(15) *When all the Knots of the Heart here (in this life) are cleft asunder, then the mortal becomes the Deathless: up to this point proceeds the Teaching.*

Once more we have the statement, quite explicit this time, that all the outer desires that cling to the heart must be detached. This teaching is cardinal in all yoga. We sometimes find attempts made to distinguish between the 'purely negative' yoga of the Buddhists and the 'more positive' teachings of the Upanishadic schools.

[1] Wittgenstein—*Tractatus Logico-Philosophicus*.

But such a distinction is, in the end, illusory. We have already seen, that, as concerns the ultimate Goal, no really positive statement can be made, though such statements are offered as helps on the way. Here too, not the Buddha himself could have stated more clearly that it is the outgoing forces of desire that hold the soul in bondage and subject it to death and again death. The fact is that all this quest for 'a more positive way' arises from the hankering to keep some at least of our cherished desires, to achieve some sort of compromise between the naked Truth and our beloved egos.

"Kill out desire" says the *Voice of the Silence*. Desire is the cause of sorrow: with the cessation of desire the Sorrowless is attained; thus teaches the Buddha and precisely the same statement is made in our text.[1]

Faced with these clear and corrosive statements the first thing we attempt is to defend ourselves against them. Desire is part of the cosmic process; without desire there would be no life at all; does not the condemnation of desire constitute an indictment of the universe? Do not other Upanishads teach us that the One *desired* to be many? Is not the aspiration for attainment also a desire? So we go on, our minds, always the willing servants of our desires, finding plenty of reasons for denying, or at least toning down, the truth of the teaching.

Desire *is* part of the cosmic process; it *is* the force which produces manifestation; it *is* the force which produces life—and death. But this Path is the Path to Life beyond these opposites, the Path, as the Teaching tells us, to the Deathless. There is no obligation for any

---

[1] Compare also the saying of Lallā, the 14th century Kashmiri Yogini: "Slay thou desire; meditate on the nature of the Self. Abandon thou thy vain imaginings for know thou that that knowledge is rare and of great price. Yet is it near by thee; search for it not afar. It is naught but a void; and a void has become merged within the Void."

to tread it who does not feel called upon to do so, but, if we decide to tread it, we should not blind our eyes to its nature. As for the aspiration towards the Goal, it is quite true that, in us, it is mixed with desire, just as, in us, love and compassion are mixed with baser elements. As the disciple proceeds upon the Path, however, the admixture becomes less and less, until, with Attainment, it vanishes for ever, or, to put it the other way, with its vanishing, Attainment shines forth.

Incidentally, the Teachers are not offering an indictment of the universe. All things have their proper place: this is the Path of Return. He who still feels the other Path, the Path of Forthgoing, is his is invited to leave this one alone.

Another defence of our minds, when faced with this teaching, is the child's trick of extreme reaction. 'You don't want me to play in the mud; then I won't play at all.' And then the child proceeds to make itself unpleasant to all around it by adopting an attitude of stony negativity until an unwise parent says 'Oh go and do what you like.' But the cosmos is not an unwise parent and a sound box on the ear is all we are likely to get as the result of our sulky negativism on this Path. We are not being asked to dramatise a spectacular attitude of stone-like, immobile indifference but to cease from plastering *ourselves* all over the universe, to cease squirting our life-blood over all things great and small and then rushing towards them in attraction or shrinking away in disgust. As for the Life that lies beyond and that is revealed in all its beauty when the squirtings have ceased, it is a state of which the less we talk the better, in order that, as Hermes says, "we may not be calumniators," for the desire-charged language of the world is no fit medium for the expression of that Life. No doubt it is beyond all we know as life but it is no less beyond the *tāmasik* indifferentism that is what we know as death.

And in any case, what exactly is desire? Desire is a movement of the psyche towards or away from (for aversion is only the negative form of desire) some object thought of as outside itself. It is thus essentially a movement of ignorance, for there is nothing that is in truth outside the Soul. The imagination creates an image and then, following the Path of Forthgoing and projecting that image 'outside,' we strive towards it or away from it in ignorance of the fact that its true being is within the Soul. Thus arises the outer world of desirable objects and thus arises our bondage to that world. Plotinus has differentiated between the archetypal circular movement of the Heavens and the rectilinear, to-and-fro movement characteristic of physical bodies. There is, however, in us too, he says, a 'circling nature' which is Divine, for "the Soul exists in revolution around God to whom it clings in love."[1] The to-and-fro movement is the movement of desire which is to be cut off while the circling or spheric movement is the characteristic of the freed Soul that has recalled its projections and lives its own Divine life. "And this is why the All, circling as it does, is at the same time at rest."[2] To use the term Desire (which belongs to the to-and-fro movement) of the spheric movement of the All, and that is the same as saying of the Soul in its free state, is a gross·

---

[1] Plotinus: On the Heavenly Circuit. *Enneads* 2, 2.

[2] Ibid. If at this point the cry is raised that the stars do not 'really' move in circles and that they are 'really' physical bodies, it can only be replied that they *do* move on circular paths from our point of view (which is all we are concerned with, all descriptions by us having reference solely to our point of view) and that they are *not* 'really' physical bodies, whatever they may be apparently. If reality is sought it is the 'Void' alone. All else is unreal.

misuse of language. The former is refuged in or clings to the heart, as the text says, because it is from the heart that go forth the projected images which draw forth the movements. Therefore it has been said in the *Secret of the Golden Flower* : "The work on the circulation of the Light (*that is, the setting up in conscious-ness of the Divine 'circular' movement*) depends entirely on the backward-flowing movement (*the calling in of the projected desire-energy*) so that the thoughts are gathered together in the place of Heavenly Consciousness, the Heavenly Heart......Therefore, when the Light cir-culates, the powers of the whole body (*the whole psyche, rather*) arrange themselves before its throne just as when a holy king has taken possession of the capital."[1] The commentator adds that this is "the way that leads from conscious action to unconscious non-action" or, in other words, from the desire prompted actions of the ignorant to the divine action in in-action of the wise.

As regards the Knots of the Heart mentioned in verse 15, Shankara states that they are the formations of Ignorance which bind us fast by causing us to assert 'I am this body, this wealth is mine, I am happy or sorrowful.' This statement is perfectly correct but its effect upon most modern men who read it will be to suggest that the knots in question are so many false intellectual beliefs which a proper knowledge of Ve-dāntic 'metaphysics' will correct. Such a view, how-ever, is far from adequate. Intellectual beliefs are only a part, and, in some sense, one of the least impor-tant parts of the contents of the psyche. They are symptoms and not causes, for they are rooted either in the desire-nature below or in the *Buddhi* above. Let us not forget that the mind is a mirror, a tool in the hands of either the 'evil daemon' below or the 'good

[1] Italics mine.

daemon' above, or, more usually, the battlefield for
these contending forces. It is, however, a *living* battlefield, one which itself takes the side of one or other of
the combatants, assisting it by every means in
its power by altering its configurations to suit the
favoured side. No man has ever had the slightest difficulty in dealing with his intellectual opinions, modify-
ing and reversing them with the utmost ease—*provided
he really wished to*. From its own point of view, and
only from that point of view, the mediaeval Roman
Catholic church was quite correct in holding that a
man who refused to exchange his 'heretical' beliefs
for the dogmas of the church was possessed by a devil,
only we should add that in truth that devil, or rather
daemon, was very often higher than all the angels of
orthodoxy. Intellectual beliefs are in fact flags waving
in the wind, whether that wind be the changeable dust-
laden winds of the earth's surface or the pure and
steadily driving tides of higher regions. Such flags
serve a useful purpose in indicating the direction of
the wind but no more, and, as the old proverb has it,
a man convinced against his will is of the same opinion
still. We believe what we want to believe, or rather,
what something in us wishes us to believe, and what
that something is, whether a mocking spirit or a beneficent God, will depend on our general psychic condition rather than on any purely intellectual considerations. Hence the sterility of mere courses of 'metaphysical' study, Vedāntik or other. The actual Knots
of the Heart are something far deeper and more difficult to untie than any mere intellectual beliefs.

There is another school of yogis who practise what
is known as *Laya Yoga* (a misleading term since all yoga
is *laya yoga*[1]) or more popularly *Kuṇḍalinī Yoga*. This

---

[1]*Laya* means absorption or merging of one principle in another.

school, which is a branch of the *Hatha Yoga*, works primarily on the physical body. On the principle 'as
above so below', they find all the higher principles
manifested in that body and seek by physical means to
act upon them there. Thus, for example, the union
of the higher *Manas* and the *Buddhi* is localised in the
Ajñā chakra between the eyebrows. The seven principles or levels of being are represented in a special
sense in the seven 'Lotuses' or centres, five of which
are in the spine. Through the centre of the latter runs
the *Sushumnā* Path. This last, conceived as a sort of
subtle nerve or channel is a physical manifestation of
the Middle Path, and, like the latter, runs straight
between two interdependent extremes, the lunar and
solar paths known as *Iḍā* and *Pingalā* respectively.
The Power, the one Power that manifests in all life, is
held to reside in the centre at the base of the spine in
the form of the Goddess *Kuṇḍalinī*, the Coiled One.
Thence by a technique consisting in the main of pos-
tures designed to bring pressure upon the nerves and
of very special breathing processes, into the theory of
which we cannot go here, she is led up the *Sushumnā*
Path to the so-called Thousand Petalled Lotus in the
head where *Samādhi* is attained. On this path three
Knots situated at the centres corresponding to the navel,
heart and eye-brows and known as the Knots of *Brahmā*, *Vishnu* and *Rudra* respectively are to be pierced.
After piercing the last of these the yogi proceeds
to the Abode of *Brahman* in the Thousand Petalled
Lotus.

The above is not intended as an exposition of this
yoga (for which indeed the present writer is not competent) nor is this the place to offer any criticism of it,
beyond saying that its chief attraction appears to be in
the vividness and the sense of concrete reality that
arises through the pre-occupation with physical pro-

cesses and at least quasi-physical sensations.[1] It is
also in this that its danger lies.   It offers little to coun-
teract our already excessive tendency to think of the
physical as the only real, at least in any vivid sense of
the word, and of only too many of its followers it is
true that what begins with the body ends there also.
That which commences with abnormal physiological
practices is only too apt to end at mere abnormal psychic powers.   Actually this brief outline has been given
because this verse and also the subsequent one are sometimes interpreted in this sense and it is important to
realise that such a view, though true within its limitations, is only an aspect of a much wider truth.   The
gross body and its subtle counterpart are only the
lowest concretisations of the total psychic being and it
is therefore to the psyche as a whole that we should
direct our attention, for it is there and not in the spine,
gross or subtle, that the fundamental Knots are found.
If, however, our excursion into *Haṭha Yoga* has given
rise to any sense that we are dealing with something
far more real than mere intellectual opinions our time
has not been wasted.

Let us return, however, to the point of view of
Rāja Yoga which, making use only of a few simple
physical preliminaries in order to clear the table as it

[1] Those who are interested in this yoga are referred to works
such as the *Varāha Upaniṣad* and to Arthur Avalon's elaborate
work entitled *'The Serpent Power'*.   In the last named book we read
—"When the Yoga is complete, the Yogi sits rigid in the posture selected and the only trace of warmth to be found in the whole
body is at the crown of the head where the Shakti is united with
Shiva. Those therefore who are sceptical can easily verify the
facts, should they be fortunate enough to find a successful Yogi
who will let them see him at work. They may observe his ecstasies
and the coldness of the body which is not present in what is called
the *Dhyāna Yogi*, or a Yogi operating by meditation only." Quite
so.

were, starts its work directly upon the mind which is the master-key of the whole process. The mind, as befits its central position, is to be trained to perform two functions, to control the senses below and to be controlled by the *Buddhi* above. The average man's mind is itself dragged hither and thither by the unruly horses of sense. On such a mind the *Buddhi* can only manifest in the form of an all-controlling fate whose dark compulsion is the inevitable counterpart of such irresponsible, sense-directed careering. Yoga is balance; he who would command must also obey and it is only by submitting itself to the commands of the *Buddhi* in all matters, by listening at all times to the Inner Voice, the voice of the Cosmic Harmony, or *Rita*, that the mind can gain the power of imposing its commands upon the senses. Then and then only can the process of *laya* be achieved and in the words of our text, the senses be merged in *Manas*, *Manas* in *Buddhi*, *Buddhi* in the Great Self and that in the Peace beyond. It is that ascent that is the fundamental, the archetypal Ascent of the Coiled One, an ascent of which all processes taking place in the spine or elsewhere are but outward manifestations, partial expressions on their own limited scale. Water the root of the tree and the whole tree will flourish. On that Middle Path of the Spirit's ascent there are three main Knots which have to be pierced, or rather untied, which untying may, as the *Haṭha yogis* truly say, involve considerable pain and even danger. The first of them is the Knot of *Brahmā*, the Knot which ties the Light of the Spirit to the sense world in general and the physical body in particular, making us say 'I am this body.' As long as we identify ourselves with physical forms, so long we share the inevitable fate of those forms, birth and death.

The second Knot is the Knot of *Vishṇu*, that by

which we are bound to the desire world, the world of feeling, and on account of which we say, in Shankara's words, 'I am happy or I am sorrowful,' and then proceed to move towards or away from the fancied causes of our happiness or sorrow in desire or aversion.

The third, the tightest Knot of all, is the knot of the mind, that which binds the Spirit to the world of thought, the rooting place and ultimate fortress of separate self-hood. All things may pass and be taken from me but in my thoughts I live for ever. Here is my self, my ultimate monad, unique, aeonian, the icy Pole-star of the universe, the diamond pivot on which all else revolves, hard with a diamond's cold and gleaming fire.

These are the three great Knots symbolised (from one point of view at least) by the triply knotted sacred thread which the Sanyāssi offers up in the fire of renunciation. They are the Knots which bind together the whole universe as we know it, not the divine and harmonious Cosmos of unity above, but the sorrowful and weary world of separateness below. All compounded things, said the Buddha, are full of sorrow. These are the knots that bring about the compounding, the triple cement that holds together our sorry dwelling. The first cement is of mud and can be washed away by water, the second is harder and must be loosened by the pointed iron of the mind while the third is the hardest of all, a secret invisible cement that can only be removed by the fire of Spirit, by burning, as the alchemists said, "in well-regulated fire." Only *Rudra* Himself in the form of *Kālāgni*, the World-destroying Fire, can dissolve the final Knot, the Knot of *Rudra*. By the *Ātman* itself is the *Ātman* to be attained. In that glowing Fire all that is mortal is consumed; that which was imprisoned in the husk of mortality re-assumes its naturally Deathless nature; the Gold of the Philoso-

phers shines in its own bright radiance. In the words
of the Buddha :—

> "O Builder, thou art seen, never again shalt thou
>   build house for me,
> Broken are all thy beams, shattered thy ridge-pole.
> My mind is set on the Uncompounded; extinguish-
>   ed are desires."

A description of the process at this stage, the
stage of dissolving the third Knot in the Centre
between the eyebrows, is given in the *Shaṭ chakra
nirūpaṇam* or *Description of the Six Centres* as follows:—
"Having closed the House which hangs without
Support, that is known through service of the Supreme
Guru, and, by repeated practice, dissolving the mind
in that abode of bliss, the yogi sees within the middle of
that space starry sparks of fire distinctly shining. Thereafter he sees the light (of the *Atman*) glowing between
Heaven and Earth like a flaming lamp, like the newly
risen sun. It is in this place that the Divine Being
becomes manifest in full power, imperishable, knowing
no decay, as in the Region of Sun, Moon and Fire."[1]

The House hanging without Support is of course
the mind which has been isolated from all worldly
connections and corresponds to the sealed Hermetic
vessel in which the alchemical 'Solution' took place.
The sparks are the lightning-like flashes, the preliminary perceptions which herald the rising of the mystic
Sun in all its fulness.

A parallel description in the form of an allegory is
contained in an old alchemical tract which describes
how a bride and bridegroom who are also brother and
sister are sealed up in a transparent chamber and warm-
ed with a gentle but prolonged heat. The first thing

[1] Ibid verses 36, 37.

that happens is that they rush into each other's arms where the bridegroom dissolves in fervent love and dies, followed shortly after by the bride. Thus only 'Water' remains but out of that Water, by further heating, arises once more the bride, now a Queen who says "I was great and became small; but now after I became humble I was raised to be a Queen of many realms." Then comes the manifestation of many marvellous Marriage Vestures and lastly the resurrection of the Bridegroom, now "a great and mighty King in all his power and glory, and there was nothing like him."[1] The exact correspondence of these two accounts should be obvious to any one who has followed all that has gone before.

"Up to this point proceeds the Teaching." Beyond this stage no further instructions can be given. The disciple has become one with the Inner Guru and must find within himself the knowledge necessary for proceeding further. "The Guru's instructions are to go above the *Ājñā Chakra,* but no special directions are given," for after this *Chakra* has been pierced, the *Sādhaka* can, and indeed must, reach the *Brahmasthāna* or Abode of *Brahman* unaided and by his own effort. "Above, the relationship of Guru and Disciple ceases."[2]

It may be as well to remind Western readers that the *Ājñā Chakra* referred to is the centre between the two eyes and is the dwelling of the Inner Guru whence issue His commands (*ājñā*). This is the 'place' where the Tāntrik tradition of *Laya Yoga* localises the above-described transformation but it will also be well to remember that it is a 'place' which is quite off the map

---

[1] A Golden Treatise about the Philosopher's Stone, translated in *Secret Symbols of the Rosicrucians.*

[2] *The Serpent Power* by Arthur Avalon.

of any anatomist. The two eyes between which it lies are only in a very limited sense the two eyes which confront us in our mirrors and, as Hermes states; "This is, my son, Rebirth,—no more to look on things from body's viewpoint (a thing three ways in space extended)." Rather the disciple has passed right through himself "into a Body that can never die"; hence his subsequent exclamation "I have had my former compounded form dismembered for me. I am no longer touched, yet I have touch; I have dimension too, and yet I am a stranger to them now."[1]

Beyond this there can be no teaching. "It is written that for him who is on the threshold of divinity no law can be framed, no guide exist. Yet to enlighten the disciple the final struggle may be thus expressed: Hold fast to that which has neither substance nor existence. Listen only to the Voice which is soundless. Look only on That which is invisible alike to the inner and the outer sense."[2]

The two verses which follow are in no sense further teaching but, as it were, after-thoughts concerning what has gone before.

(16) *A hundred and one are the subtle channels of the heart: of them one extends upwards to the crown of the head. Having gone up by that, one goes to Deathlessness; the others are for going forth differently.*

The word *nāḍi* which has been translated as subtle channel literally means a tube or hollow pipe. It is sometimes translated as artery, vein or nerve as is also the word *hitā* which is used in similar contexts in some other Upanishads. Such a rendering however has

[1] *The Secret Sermon.* Hermetic Corpus, 13.
[2] *Light on the Path.*

given rise to a good deal of misunderstanding. The hundred and one (a round number of course, elsewhere given as seventy-two thousand.)[1] *nāḍis* are neither the arterial-venous system nor yet the nervous system, at least, not in the primary sense, though both those networks are no doubt connected with and manifestations of the archetypal *nāḍi* system. It is true that the *Haṭha Yogi*, as we have already observed, works on and makes use of the nervous system, but that is by correspondence in the same way that control of ordinary breathing is undertaken in order to control the subtle *Prāṇa* and through that the still subtler *Manas*. It cannot be too often insisted that the real *nāḍi* system with all its associated 'lotuses' or *chakras* is fundamentally a psychic system. The 'subtle channels' are the network of paths along which psychic and not physical energy is organised and transmitted, which is why they are said to be filled with an essence which is white, blue, yellow, green and red,[2] colours which are the same as those in the mystical Sun. During sleep the *Jīva*, the point-like individual centre or psychic focus, is said to wander about in that system of many-coloured channels.

The system as a whole is in fact the mystic Net which is lowered into the waters of the Bitter Sea, the Net to which Christ referred when he promised to make his disciples 'Fishers of Men', and which only appears as the nervous system when seen through the highly refracting waters of the depths.[3]

---

[1] *Brihadāranyaka Upanishad*, 2, 1, 19.

[2] *Brihadāranyaka Upanishad*, 4, 3, 20.

[3] There are many interesting references to this symbolic net in ancient mystical literature. In *Shwetāshwatara Upanishad*, Ishwara is termed the Wielder of the Net, and in the Egyptian *Book of the Dead* (Chapter 153A, Budge), under the vignette of a net, occur the following interesting words: "Hail, thou 'God who

Chapter VI

Just as, however, in the physical nervous system
there is one nerve, the spinal cord, which runs from the
base of the trunk to its summit, the head, so is there in
the psyche one subtle Path known as the Royal Path,
the Path of *Brahman* and the *Sushumnā*,[1] which, as the
Tāntriks say, contains Sun, Moon and Fire, and, which
runs from the depths of our being to the very summit:

> "On it, they say, are white and blue, yellow and
> green and red,
> That was the Path found by *Brahmā*, by it goes
> the Knower of the *Brahman*."[2]

It is in fact the famous Middle Path which mediates
between the two extremes, between the hot Solar Path
of the right hand and the cold Lunar Path of the left.
All the positive phenomena of life, all the sons of the
Sun in fact, have shadows which are Daughters of the
Moon. None can one-sidedly stretch forth a bright hand
to seize, without a dark hand being stretched forth to
seize the seizer. All actions have their equal and opposite reactions and therefore, as Heracleitus taught, all
things pass into their opposites. This is the ever-moving Breath of Life, the Breath that holds the universe in
being. Therefore the yogi checks his Breathing while
as Shankara says, "fools merely hold their noses."

lookest behind' thee (*manas* united with *buddhi*), thou 'God who
hast gained the mastery over thy heart,' I go a-fishing with the
cordage of the (Net) 'Uniter of the Earth' and of him that makest
way through the earth. Hail, ye Fishers who have given birth to
your own Fathers (*manas* in which the Divine Birth has taken
place)."
   [1] The *Sushumnā* does not primarily mean the spinal cord or any
other physiological nerve. Primarily it is the name of the chief
among the seven mystical Rays of the Sun, the one which shines
on the Moon and as such is the Path which unites Sun and Moon
in the Mystic Marriage.
   [2] *Brihadāranyaka Upanishad*, 4, 4, 9.

But "Yoga is balance." Between Sun and Moon there is a neutral point, a *Laya* centre which is the fulcrum Archimedes sought from which to move the world. Not only between Sun and Moon but between every bright, right-handed, Solar phenomenon on any level of being and its dark, left-handed, Lunar shadow, this central point of balance, the point of *laya* or dissolution exists and is to be found by the yogi. When he stands balanced upon that Point he is free from the Pair of Opposites and, as he passes through it, the Sun and Moon, as represented in that particular Pair, come together in the Centre and are no more. The *Sushumnā* or 'Middle Path' is the line that joins all such points, the unique central path in the very midst of our being. As the yogi travels along it the whole universe falls into dissolution behind him as did the Mystic Bridge behind the leaping feet of Galahad. All other paths are mere side-tracks leading in various directions to various partial aims each of which has its compensating shadow. This alone is the unique, the shadowless Path, the Path that leads from death to Deathlessness, the Swan's Path through the Void that leads to Bliss.

The following quotations from the Sayings of Lallā, a fourteenth century Kashmiri yogini who had actually travelled this Path, are added as being incomparably more vivid than anything the present writer could say:

"With passionate longing, I Lallā, went forth;
Searching and seeking, Day and Night vanished
    for me ;
Then I saw in my own House a Wise man;
When I seized hold of him that was the moment
    of the rising of my star.

"O Guru ! O Supreme Lord ! Explain to me

the inner meaning known to thee:
There are two breathings which arise from the
vital centre.[1]
Why is one breathing 'cold,' the other 'hot' ?"

The Guru's answer to this question is too technical
to be given here but later she writes:—

"My Guru uttered but one instruction, 'from without enter thou into the inmost.'
And that became for me a guiding principle, a
mantra;
Therefore naked I began to dance.

"I closed the doors and windows of the House of
my body;
I seized the thief of my *Prāṇas* and controlled my
breathing;
I bound him in the dark cell of my heart
And with the whip of *OM* I flayed him.

"I, Lallā, entered through the door of the Jasmine
Garden.
There, O wonderful, I saw Shiva united with his
Shakti;
There I dissolved myself in the Lake of the Water
of Life;
Now what can harm me who, even while living,
shall be as dead.

"Eagerly seeking I came from the inmost recess
into the Moonlight.
Eagerly seeking I came, like being joined to like.
Thou alone, O Dweller in the Waters, Thou alone!

[1] Literally 'the City of the Bulb,' a technical term of Yoga.

All this is Thou alone! What are these shinings-forth?

"When by yoga practice the outspread universe
has become absorbed in that which is above it,
Its varied qualities are fused within the Void of
Space.
When that Void has also dissolved, then but the
Sorrowless remains;
This is the teaching to thee, O *Brāhman*."[1]

(17) *The Thumb-like Puruṣha, the Inner Soul, is ever
seated in the heart of all beings. Him one should patiently
draw forth from one's body like a reed from its outer sheath.
Know him to be the Pure, the Deathless. Yes, know him to
be the Pure, the Deathless.*

In conclusion, the essence of the whole yoga is
stated once again in the simplest terms as if to remind
the disciple that all the complicated details hinted at in
the previous verse are only one way of describing the
process. Such separate descriptions are not to be taken
as being so many separate yogas. There is only one
yoga which, not being a process of the sense world, cannot be described in direct terms, for "our enquiry obliges
us to use terms not strictly applicable,"[2] but only in symbols of which there are a rich variety suited to different
temperaments. To some an intricate symbolism such as
that of the '*Kuṇḍalinī yoga*' is felt to be oppressive with its
weight of detail. To other types it is just that richness
of detail that is helpful since it gives rise in their minds
to a feeling of reality, of dealing with actual things by

[1] The above translation has been made with the help of
Grierson and Barnett's.

[2] *Plotinus*, 6, 8, 13.

actual processes.

In all cases the essence is the same. The inner Self, the Centre of our whole being, the secret source of power which dwells in the heart of the psyche, is poised between two worlds, the 'light-wrapped' region above and the 'dark-rayed, gloom-wrapped' land below. The process of birth is the self-identification of that central soul with the latter and with a physical body in particular, that physical body which to the Orphic Initiates was known as the Tomb.

The process of yoga is the withdrawal of that projection, the gradual severing of that bond of identification, and the consequent return to the regions of Light which are the Soul's true home. This is the "flight to the beloved Fatherland" of Plato and Plotinus and this the withdrawal or separation of the Thumb-like *Purusha* mentioned in our text. "Many times has it happened; lifted out of the body into myself; becoming external to all other things and self-encentred; beholding a marvellous beauty; then more than ever assured of community with the loftiest order."[1]

This withdrawal is symbolised in our text as being like the extraction of the central core of a reed from its outer sheath[2] but this again is only description and should not set us thinking in terms of spatial movements of 'astral' bodies. "The Soul's 'separate place'" as Plotinus says, "is simply its not being in Matter; that is, its not being united with it" and the *Chaldæan Oracles* say plainly: "believe thyself to be out of the body and thou art." It is necessary to add, however, that such 'believing' is not the pious wishing that commonly pas-

[1] *Plotinus*, 4, 8, 1.
[2] It is interesting to note that the type of reed mentioned was one used for making arrows, which reminds us of the famous arrow of the Soul that is to be shot into the heart of the *Brahman* (*Muṇḍaka Upanishad*, 2, 2, 3 and 4).

ses as such and, which in fact, is seldom more than a game of 'makebelieve.' It is by believing that we find ourselves embodied and the 'belief' which liberates from embodiment must be one of equal power and vividness if it is to be effective. Such a belief is only possible to a mind which has been purified by long and arduous preliminary training in yoga. It is only in such a mind that the Knowledge of the *Buddhi* can be reflected, such reflection being, as we have said before, the true and only real faith.

Poised as it is between the Desire-principle below and the *Buddhi* above there are only two types of reflection or faith possible, according to which way the mental mirror is turned. If below, then the reflection is inevitably one of something outside the self, an external world which in the last resort must be one of 'dead' matter, to which the soul is bound by chains of desire. If, on the other hand, the mind is turned towards the above, the reflection will be of an inner world of light and harmony which there pervades the soul with freedom and bliss.

These are the only two real faiths, faith in the dark and demonic enchantress of desire, and faith in the divine Goddess of the Wisdom. All that lies between is a misty mid-region of phantasy, in which there can be no certainty and no resolute action in either direction, since, in it, every light has its shadow and every belief its compensating doubt gnawing at its heart.

This is borne out by ordinary experience in the world in which we see that only two types of men are really resolute, certain and sure, both of themselves and of the world around them. One is the materialist, the convinced believer in matter, who, though indeed making no claim to universal knowledge, is yet convinced that, by following the principles of science, such knowledge will in the end be attained. The other is the believer in spirit, the follower of the inner not the outer light; he too moves in the world with the same certainty of conviction as does the materialist.

These are the two extremes. Between them are found the many who are lower than either, the few who are above both. The first class comprises all the dwellers in the realm of muddle, scientists whose hearts are gnawed by secret superstitions, clay-footed idealists whose thoughts are beautiful but actions ugly. The second class comprises the perfected Yogis, who, as the Gita tells us, are but a tiny few even among the few who strive for yoga. They are the knowers of the double Knowledge, Lords of the Double-Axe, masters of both the Cosmic Tides; they who "by knowledge of the Ignorance, passing beyond death, by knowledge of the Wisdom, gain the Immortal."[1]

There are thus two Ways, the dark Way of Matter and the bright Way of Spirit. Between them both are two mid-regions, the region of muddle and the region of Mastery. In the very Centre of all stands the All-inclusive, the Supreme, the stainless Eternal, beyond Spirit and Matter, beyond Wisdom and Ignorance, beyond Mastery and muddle and yet including all, the ultimate Thatness of which we must perforce be silent.

Returning therefore to that of which speech is possible let us resolutely draw forth the Inner Soul from its various bodily sheaths, the sheath of sensations, the sheath of feelings and the inmost sheath of thoughts. The task is a difficult one, but what man has done man can do again, and with patient resolution, the Inner Soul, if firmly seized with the grasp of a discriminating self-identification, emerges from its wrappings clean and straight like the reed to which the text compares it.

[1] *Ishopanishad*, II.

That, it is true, is not the final End, for as the symbolism again reminds us, the Soul thus freed is still a thing-in-itself, 'pure and deathless' but still separate from other Souls. The Path leads on beyond all separateness, beyond all self-existing monads whatsoever, but the further reaches of the Way are, as Hermes says, "Not taught." The Journey through the Darkness is ended; only the Journey through the Light remains. Within that Light which now surrounds it, the Soul must seek the power and wisdom for its further self-annihilating progress: as our Upanishad itself observes, "Up to this point proceeds the Teaching." The rest is Silence.

(18) *Then Nachiketas, having obtained this Knowledge, taught by Death, and the complete instructions of Yoga, attaining the* Brahman *became free from all passion, free from death. So also may any other who thus knows the nature of the* Ātman.

"These things, O Asclepius, will appear true if thou understand them; but if thou understand them not, incredible. For to understand is to believe; not to believe is not to understand."[1]

So, in truth may we. In the words of the *Emerald Tablet*: "What I have to say about the masterpiece of the Alchemical Art, the Solar Work, is ended."

[1] Hermes Trismegistus.

Made in the USA
Columbia, SC
21 July 2019